AF 141139

Tucholsky Wagner Zola Scott Sydow Freud Schlegel
Turgenev Wallace Fonatne
Twain Walther von der Vogelweide Fouqué Friedrich II. von Preußen
Weber Freiligrath Frey
Fechner Fichte Weiße Rose von Fallersleben Kant Ernst Frommel
Richthofen
Hölderlin
Engels Fielding Eichendorff Tacitus Dumas
Fehrs Faber Flaubert
Eliasberg Ebner Eschenbach
Feuerbach Maximilian I. von Habsburg Fock Eliot Zweig
Ewald Vergil
Goethe Elisabeth von Österreich London
Mendelssohn Balzac Shakespeare Dostojewski Ganghofer
Lichtenberg Rathenau Doyle Gjellerup
Trackl Stevenson Tolstoi Hambruch
Mommsen Thoma Lenz Hanrieder Droste-Hülshoff
Dach Verne von Arnim Hägele Hauff Humboldt
Reuter Rousseau Hagen Hauptmann Gautier
Karrillon Garschin Defoe Baudelaire
Damaschke Descartes Hebbel
Hegel Kussmaul Herder
Wolfram von Eschenbach Dickens Schopenhauer Rilke George
Bronner Darwin Melville Grimm Jerome
Campe Horváth Aristoteles Bebel Proust
Bismarck Vigny Barlach Voltaire Federer Herodot
Gengenbach Heine
Storm Casanova Tersteegen Grillparzer Georgy
Chamberlain Lessing Langbein Gilm Gryphius
Brentano Lafontaine
Strachwitz Claudius Schiller Kralik Iffland Sokrates
Katharina II. von Rußland Bellamy Schilling Raabe Gibbon Tschechow
Gerstäcker
Löns Hesse Hoffmann Gogol Wilde Gleim Vulpius
Luther Heym Hofmannsthal Klee Hölty Morgenstern
Roth Heyse Klopstock Kleist Goedicke
Luxemburg Puschkin Homer Mörike
La Roche Horaz Musil
Machiavelli Kierkegaard Kraft Kraus
Navarra Aurel Musset Moltke
Nestroy Marie de France Lamprecht Kind Kirchhoff Hugo
Laotse Ipsen Liebknecht
Nietzsche Nansen Ringelnatz
Marx Lassalle Gorki Klett Leibniz
von Ossietzky May vom Stein Lawrence Irving
Petalozzi Knigge
Platon Pückler Michelangelo Kock Kafka
Sachs Poe Liebermann
de Sade Praetorius Mistral Zetkin Korolenko

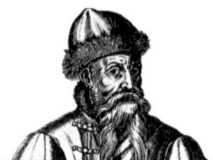
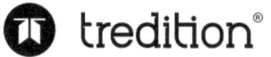

Valere Aude Dare to Be Healthy, Or, The Light of Physical Regeneration

Louis Dechmann

Imprint

This book is part of the TREDITION CLASSICS series.

Author: Louis Dechmann
Cover design: toepferschumann, Berlin (Germany)

Publisher: tredition GmbH, Hamburg (Germany)
ISBN: 978-3-8491-7409-5

www.tredition.com
www.tredition.de

TABLE OF CONTENTS

DEDICATION

To you of that great voiceless multitude,

"THE PEOPLE"—

You whose bewildered cry is still for light; whose silent tragedy our well beloved Longfellow could so well portray:

"O suffering sad humanity!
O ye afflicted ones, who lie
Steeped to the lips in misery,
Longing, and yet afraid to die,
Patient, though sorely tried!"

To you and your needs this brief epitome of a coming greater work is given as a fitting Christmas offering—

"LET THERE BE LIGHT!"

It is the cry which despairing, deluded humanity, in the darkness of its frenzied ignorance, has flung back hopelessly to heaven since first the spirit of an Infinite Intelligence brooded upon the race. It is the appeal of man's immortal unity to the All-Father, from age to age, for knowledge sufficient for its hourly needs, since ever, back in the far dim ages of the earth, primeval man, beetle-browed, furtive and fashioned fearsomely, first felt the faint vibration of a Soul; and, like an awakened giant, that chief of human faculties, a Mind took form which, pressing on along the uncertain way, has scaled the giddy heights of knowledge where genius, enthroned, does battle with an envious world of shams and greed and venal prejudice. Led by the resistless pulse of power it follows still that "banner with a strange device: Excelsior!";—for, ever onward yet it wends its way where'er the devious pathway trends, whose troubled, varied course is time, whose bourne is in eternity.

But where seek we, then, the answer to a cry so shrill, that smites the high face of heaven from a world in pain?

Shall we seek it where false learning leads us in the quest?—Ah no.

It comes, not in the crash of Sinai's thunders with the rockings of a riven sphere, as in the allegoric stories of a puerile past.

Softly it falls—yes, almost fearfully—from the fervid lips of some lone world-neglected persecuted man—some patient toil-worn son of science, whom Genius loves to call her own—though, haply, to the schools, to fortune and to fame unknown. One whose transcendent, superconscious mind has dared, Prometheus-like, to snatch from heaven the fire of the immortal gods and offer it in benefits to all mankind.

Thrice happy he upon the sensory surface of whose open mind such seeds of knowledge and of wisdom fall, and happy the land where one and all may dare to warm chill hands and hearts before its sacred flame; that halcyon land, the Ultima Thule of our fond imaginings, wherein true freedom reigns; wherein the legalized tyranny of the chartered libertines of a so-called learned profession shall be finally relegated, in common cause to the limbo of a sordid and degraded past. For these are they who seek to maintain a strangle-hold on science, who paralyze the arm of individual research and, even in this advancing age, still block the path of progress and of peace, of universal freedom and equality of intellect, to all beyond the narrow limits of their own elect.

Thus then, to the free fraternity of the open mind I dedicate this brief resumé of the product of long years of study and of toil, steadfastly believing that therein is found the missing dimension for their urgent need, suited alike to all who hold that to maintain the health of body and of mind is a worthy object for enlightened man. To you, mothers of the land, who recognize your duty, towards God and to the State, to rear your children healthy, strong and good to look upon. To all whose keener common-sense looks upon Nature, the

Creator, as logically therefore, the healing power also. To all endowed with wit to understand the obvious truth that, not by poisonous drugs is healing wrought, but by such reasonable help as man's intelligence can afford, to second nature's effort to that end; and further, that, in order to achieve success, it is useless to attack, suppress or remove the symptoms of disease by force of drugging or the knife, whilst the *cause* of the evil is left untouched, unthought of, and, too frequently, unknown. Truth and reason alike proclaim: remove the cause and the symptom *must* disappear.

To all, then, to whom the ever blessed triad of health, hope, and happiness on earth, are dear, the sanctity of child-life and the improvement of the race; and especially to those whose clearer mental vision can grasp the stupendous fact of eternal Universal Unity — the oneness with that mighty Primal Cause, the great Life Principle, immanent and active throughout all nature; can grasp and assimilate the idea that everything that has life is, each in its separate form and degree, but a medium through which the Infinite Universal Source of Life — that vast, ineffable power which we, blindly, designate as God — or Good — seeks expression in the scheme of evolution whose aim sublime is pure perfection, as its ultimate, attainable, though far off goal. Directed and attracted by an intelligence we call divine, it is a hope, instinct with ability, implanted by that Power in the soul of man, as patent in his ceaseless struggle upward toward the light of fuller knowledge; it is a power, restricted, only in degree, by that individual sense of human limitations fostered by false prophets and grounded in the vitals of the race.

To you all, this brief precis is presented, as a guide, with the author's benediction, coupled with the fervent hope that, reading the scientific deductions and precepts therein contained you, too, may see Regeneration's Light and seeing, may

"Dare to be Healthy."

LOUIS DECHMANN,

Christmas, 1918. Seattle, Wash.

"Dare to be Healthy"

FORE-WORD

To the Reader:

The volume, shortly to be published, and to which the ensuing pages are designed to serve the purpose of stepping-stone or forecast, has been compiled for the purpose of placing before the public the experiences of thirty-five full years of my life as a biologist and physiological chemist, devoted to the sifting and solution of vital problems of health and eugenics and in the practice of the resultant knowledge of the laws of life discovered in the course of my research.

I would beseech you, in your own vital interest, to peruse these pages thoughtfully and with an open mind. There are throughout America already, thousands of steadfast disciples who are daily reaping the benefits of the teachings contained therein; and I would that you also may be added to that goodly multitude, to enjoy together with them the best advantages emanating from systematic study along the most advanced lines of modern thought and science. The facts are correlated and simply expressed with the earnest desire to bring within the scope of the layman the good that may accrue. It is, however, not for the laymen alone that this work is undertaken, but for unprofessional and professional alike, be he medical student or practitioner or other interested person; for to each and all I present herein the best that a lifetime of research has enabled me to wring from nature's secret store for the betterment and conservation of human life and the help of human kind.

In the development of my movement I have formulated a system under which all may participate in the benefits of my message, though possibly prevented by circumstances in some cases from coming within direct personal contact with myself.

This system comprises the following:

The "Dare to be Healthy" Club.

The "Dare to be Healthy" Lecture Course.

The "Dare to be Healthy" Hygienic Dietetic Course.

Full particulars regarding these will appear at a subsequent point in this prospectus.

LOUIS DECHMANN.

INTRODUCTION

> "... Argentea proles,
> Auro deterior, fulvo pretiosior aere."
>
> (Ovid)
>
> Succeeding times a silver age behold
> Excelling brass, but more excelled by Gold.

Hessiod, in his celebrated distribution of mankind, divides the species into three orders of intellect.

"The first place," says he, "belongs to him who can, by his own powers, discern what is fit and right, and penetrate to the remoter motives of action.

"The second place is claimed by him who is willing to hear instruction and can perceive right and wrong when they are shown to him by another; — but he who hath neither acuteness nor docility — who can neither find the way by himself, nor will be led by others, is a wretch without use or value."

"You are seeking truth," quoth Adalbert von Chamisso, *"Remember that the world clings more firmly to superstition than to faith,"* — or, to borrow expression from an equally inspired source, — remember that perverse humanity rarely fails to favour, rather, what Shakespeare terms *"The seeming truth which cunning times put on to entrap the wisest."*

Courageous, then, must be the knight who sets his lance in rest to tilt against the windmills of the world.

Nevertheless, although the truth is still banned as "heterodox" by common consent — or tacit connivance — an attitude patent to commercial instincts in view of the cataclysm which must naturally ensue, with deadly results to the vested interests of orthodoxy, so soon as the long-trusted barriers of plausible and pretentious mystery and importance shall be swept away by the rising tide of popular indignation. When the masses become educated to discriminate between truth and falsehood and thus shall come into their rights, then and not till then, will the dawn of physical salvation break.

Still, I maintain, there are, and have been all along the way, eminent medical men of high intelligence, who, unlike the drones of the medical hive, have dared to think for themselves and have even dared to speak their thoughts.

Thus, for instance, spoke Sir William W. Gull, Physician to her late Majesty Queen Victoria: "Having passed the period of the gold-headed cane and horsehair wig, we dare hope to have also passed the days of pompous emptiness; and furthermore, *we can hope that nothing will be considered unworthy the attention of physicians which contributes to the saving of life.*"

Again, an authority of the first rank, Prof. Oesterlin, says in his noted work on the Materia Medica:

"The studious physician of our century will hardly expect to accomplish by force, through some strange drug or other, that which only nature can bring about when assisted by all the rational accessories of hygiene and dietetics.

Nature alone can furnish the beneficient means, sufficient for all needs,"—which the science of medicine never has afforded and never can.

As we survey the civilization of our age and its medical science, we see, on the one hand, the crude superstitions of the masses, the subtler superstitions of the educated classes; gross materialism, bewildering Darwinism, pessimism, and degenerate political economy; on the other hand, unmitigated quackery and cupidity, with its weight of oppression on humanity,—everywhere confusion instead of harmony.

Very surely,—and perhaps more speedily than we think—a reaction will come, when our present degenerate system of medical subterfuge—misnamed science—will have passed away, to be replaced by accredited methods of natural healing consistent with the dignity of an enlightened, self-respecting people.

"Ignorance is the curse of God:
Knowledge the wing wherewith we fly to heaven"

(Shakespeare)

THE HYGIENIC-DIETETIC METHOD OF HEALING

Biology, the Science of life, has developed under my hand that system of natural healing which I practice, in common with some of the most successful physicians on the continents of Europe and America.

Although based upon the same biological laws, their systems of therapy—or healing—differ materially from one another. My system is entirely my own, developed during the last thirty-five years to that degree of perfection it has attained today.

I am, naturally, honestly proud of the success achieved during this strenuous period, yet am I still as anxiously imbued as ever with the spirit and habit of research which is now directed to the endeavour to further simplify my method of treatment, by further discoveries in the realm of that most abstruse of the sciences, *Physiological Chemistry*.

In this baffling but wonderful domain I am inspired by the ambitious hope that some, at any rate, of the many unsolved problems of the Science of Life may yet give up their secrets to the demand of my persistency, exerted in the interest of the well-being of humanity.

After centuries devoted by the faculty to a futile and arrogant attempt to counteract the disturbances of health, which we call diseases, in the stereotyped manner known as "orthodox;" after endless complications, infinite "specializing"—in itself a futility—and unblushing complicity with the powers that be, we find them now at length, baffled, discredited, but unashamed, cast back, discomforted, upon Mother Nature's kindly breast, their victims humbly seeking healing in simple unity from her ample store.

Based upon this firm foundation, we term the new departure the "Natural Method of Healing."

The greatest physicians of all time, from Hippocrates to our own day, were satisfied to be simply *natural* physicians. They were not satisfied to merely suppress the symptoms of suffering and to quiet the sufferer by abnormal appliances. Their higher, more ambitious aim was to reach the active source of distress—and in this they succeeded.

For, not only did they achieve where others failed, but, in addition to healing, they also *prevented the recurrence* of disease, and, more noteworthy still, they established a system of Prophylactic Therapy, which is the highest function of the healing art; namely, the *prevention of disease* by treatment *before full development*, or, in other words, the *preservation of health.*

It is not the object of this brief brochure to enter into the devious details which a full explanation of this practical, successful, modern method would require. It is designed merely for those who, after experiencing disappointment and failure in other directions, have had recourse, as a last alternative, to advice and assistance, from myself.

Such patients, as a rule, have heard of my method from others; have heard that it differs widely, in its frank simplicity, from the empty pomposity of the old-school "orthodox" elements, though of the principles of the old-school teaching they have really little or no conception, beyond a crude, unwholesome, fear of the unknown, consequent upon the, *very necessary*, veil of mystery with which its votaries surround themselves—a semi-superstitious sentiment inherited from a malignant past and one which does little credit to the vaunted modern civilization of today.

On this point of difference they ask for enlightenment, and naturally enquire as to the nature of both, but especially of this new hope which is held out to them as a refuge in their hour of despair.

This information it is equally my duty and my desire to give, and in the most convenient and simple form, shorn of all shroud of mystery; for my object is to educate and not to conceal.

It is my chief desire that patients should thoroughly understand the methods and principles of the New-School of Healing and should exercise their own intelligence as to its merits as compared with the old, and, being once thoroughly convinced—not by faith, or fear, or fashion, nor yet biased by the unfair influence of the false prestige of a legalized monopoly detrimental to the interest of the people—they should forthwith honestly test the new deliverance by faithfully following my advice and instruction, to their own unfailing ultimate benefit and relief.

As a labour of love towards the world in general and the people of my adopted country in particular, I have made it my duty to formulate the substance of my researches in the field of science — researches which represent the struggles of a lifetime — in a large and comprehensive work which, to the scientist as well as to the laymen, will constitute in the most detailed and complete degree a reliable guide to the conservation of health which, even now, in the immediate present, has come to be regarded not only as a scientific phase of education, but as a duty incumbent upon every citizen. Should sickness supervene, as well it may sometimes, despite all reasonable precaution, the knowledge and instructions contained therein are sufficient, if closely followed, to prevent, for the most part, the serious consequences of disease and to afford the patient the necessary enlightenment to enable him to co-operate with the hygienic-dietetic physician in the task of restoring him to health and ability.

This book, entitled *"Regeneration"* or *"Dare to be Healthy,"* will consist of some three thousand or more pages. It will be published shortly; and, in the common interests of human health will I, trust, find prominent place on the book-shelf of every home whose inmates either belong to the ever increasing number of the followers of my patients, or who, by careful study of my teachings therein contained, may be finding their independent way back from the dreary depths of suffering to the glad plains of health.

In following up the general outline of the "New Regeneration" these pages will not lend themselves to the otherwise necessary encounter with what are now admitted to be the recognized errors of the, temporarily dominant, medical school, save in so far as it may be requisite to remove from the mind of the layman pernicious and antiquated ideas to which he has been long and persistently educated, or to protect those who have ceased to believe in them from the pitfalls to which, as an alternative, they may be exposed amongst the numberless unscientific, quasi-miraculous, healing cults, or the equally pernicious nostrums of the spectacular advertising medicine vendor, both of whom reap golden harvests among the ranks of the so justly disappointed and despairing people.

It is, nevertheless, an imperative duty to issue this necessary warning; namely, that the public should safeguard itself against the absurd, but possible mistakes of confusing the Legitimate Scientific School of the Hygienic Dietetic Method of Biological Healing with the nebulous cults aforesaid. There is no vestige of resemblance between them, either in thought or principle, and nothing could be more fatal and foreign to the truth.

There is one thing, and one only, which, like the rest of the community, we share with them in common, and this is that *growing spirit of profound distrust* with which all classes seem daily more and more constrained to regard the Medical Fraternity and all its ways.

It is the general knowledge of the existence of this sentiment which has called into being the present epidemic of curious cults and catholicons—due, it would appear, more to this insidious temptation to such *commercial enterprise* than to any other cause—and which form so prominent a feature throughout all sections of the community—and especially in the press—throughout the length and breadth of the land. To such, in an alarming degree, the public turns, in protest, as it were, against the tyranny and turpitude of this "learned profession," with its kindred corporations and its studied callous disregard of scientific advancement in any direction which might tend to jeopardize or reduce the profitable exercise of its own obsolete methods, its system of poisonous medicaments, and dangerous operations and anti-toxins.

There is no possible efficacy or help to be derived from other teachings, whatsoever they may be, except from those based absolutely upon the solid foundation of biological fact. Since Johannes Müller (1833) wrote the first book on physiology and its chemistry, more than a thousand so-called "Authorities" in that branch of science have tried to find some of the secrets of nature pertaining to physiology. A very few (about 10 or 12) may be named as great men who discovered certain laws and solved certain problems. But the majority added nothing to Müller's discoveries. Most of them became teachers or authors, one plagiarizing the work of the other, eulogy being very liberally distributed on all sides, but valuable deductions from the great masters, very few have been able to make, and even those were more or less suppressed by the "orthodox school." In less than half the time since 1833, i.e. 85 years, it was my good fortune to give more valuable deductions and practical applications to the student and the reader, than the mediocre talents of the "old school" were able to give.

I pretend to no miracles and expect none; nor do I arrogate to myself any so-called *super*-natural secrets or powers; I simply maintain that, aided by the erudition of the great scientists of the past and present, this system has finally been brought to a point which should rightly have been always the chief aim of Medical Science, namely, an *exact knowledge of human nature and the human organism, as it is.*

With this vital knowledge at command I have been able to successfully formulate a system for supplying the individual organism with any of the various constituents of which it may be deficient, in a manner in which it can best receive and assimilate the same, thereby maintaining a correct balance between the constituents of the blood wherein lies hidden the sole criterion of health and the fatal secret of disease.

Simple as this may sound, the way has been long and lonely until that elusive goal was reached; and, even now, in the heat of the controversy which ensues, we find ourselves sometimes in a somewhat parlous position, placed, as it were, between two fires; on the one side are those who, though not without sympathetic feeling for the well-intentioned, earnest-minded believers in the errors now being exposed, yet cast aside all scruples in the interest of humanity and truth. On the other side are those obsessed by care and compunction for these accredited practitioners who by reason of age or temperament are unable or unwilling to assimilate new ideas or to relinquish the theories of a life time in order to enter the field of competition with the men of a younger generation.

Such is the impasse before which we stand.

REGENERATION OF THE RACE

BY THE LIGHT OF BIOLOGY AIDED BY PHYSIOLOGICAL CHEMISTRY.

"For as the body is one, and hath many members, and all the members of that one body, being many, are one body:... whether one member suffer, all the members suffer with it; or one member be honoured, all the members rejoice with it."

(St. Paul, I Corinthians, XII. 12 & 26.)

"DYSAEMIA, or Impure Blood is the cause and source of disorder in all constitutional diseases. So spoke the Master. Believe it who will, that, in a nutshell, is 'the burden of my song' — the Alpha and Omega of my teaching."

(From Chapter X. "Dare to be Healthy.")

The Process of Natural Healing is the art of curing diseases by natural methods.

As natural remedies, only those may be included which stand as vital conditions in constant relation to the organism, assimilable thereby.

Among these are no poisons or chemical preparations, such as were promulgated by Paracelsus and the medicasters; for these are elements abnormal to the body, and call forth its reactionary powers, and so, being useless, they are eliminated; or, after having served an improper purpose, to *suppress* some symptom of disease, they become embedded in the tissues, there causing various forms of medicinal complication or morbid condition.

Do we not produce blood poisons enough by our irrational diet and modes of living? The human body is a microcosm — a world in minature — and as such, exists in constant interchange with universal nature.

A definite relationship exists between it and the solid, fluid and gaseous elements.

Solid food, water and air, elements of the universe, must become elements of our bodies, if relations of universal unity are to be maintained.

There must be a constant interchange of organic matter, and this inter-transmission is the cause of life, of health, and of disease; therefore, we must first of all see that the conditions of this process are uninterrupted.

Food, air, water, light, exercise, must be so provided that they condition the process of nutrition and metamorphosis.

Skin, lungs, kidneys, intestines, must always be in condition to eliminate the abnormal products of decomposition.

If then disease be a derangement of the life process, it is self-evident that disease is not confined to one organ alone, but that the whole body is diseased.

The body, thus, being in fact an indivisible unity, the treatment we employ in disease must, logically, act upon it as a united whole.

The modern school of medicine in its present, bacteria ridden frame of mind or mania, looks upon the bacillus, or microbe, as the sole cause of disease.

The cause, however, is not the bacillus, but rather the impure blood which prepares a fertile soil for the development of those destructive germs.

He who lives strictly in accordance with the rules of hygiene need not fear the bacillus, for man is not born to sickness; he creates sickness for himself by his irrational mode of living.

What does the world profit by bacteriological institutions if the people continue to live in the old sins against health and hygiene?

Man may be born with a predisposition to disease, but not with disease itself.

Our health depends entirely upon the conditions of our life.

In cases of predisposition to disease, therefore, as well as in disease itself, according to the principles of hygiene, we must employ only the hygienic and dietetic methods of treatment.

Is the medical science of the day, then, totally incompetent? You may well ask.—Have the patient studies and researches of nearly two thousand four hundred years, since the days of Hippocrates, been all in vain?

The reply lies ready to your hand, from the lips of one of the brightest scientific spirits that ever illumined this dull earth of ours with knowledge and sincerity.

In Goethe's Faust the following lines are found,—lines which sad memory brings back to the minds of many an unfortunate who, according to the dictates of the medical science of today, is pronounced incurable—a sufferer from one or other of the so-called chronic diseases—and in dire need of both physical and spiritual support.

> "I have, alas, philosophy,
> Medicine, jurisprudence too,
> And, to my cost, theology
> With ardent labour studied through,
> And here I stand with all my lore,
> Poor fool, no wiser than before"

Like Faust, such sufferers study day and night the opinions of learned doctors and follow their prescriptions with ardent zeal. The more they study, the more doctors they consult, the more rapidly does strength fail them, until at length they realize that, in spite of all their lore, they are but "poor fools, no wiser than before."

For more than two thousand years it has been, in fact, as it is to a great extent today; the physician prescribes to the best of his knowledge, medicines compounded according to certain rules dogmatically laid down in the schools.

Here we have at once the fatal mistake at a glance.

Instead of studying nature and the laws of nature, instead of using natural means to *heal disease*, they administer deadly poisons to *allay suffering*, poisons, which doubtless may be able to repress pain or to temporarily suppress the symptoms of disease; but can *never remove the cause*, which alone may rightly be called healing.

The drugs prescribed by thousands of physicians today, with but a casual acquaintance with their action, are bound by their nature to produce evils worse than the disease itself.

To cite an instance:

Physicians prescribe creosote in cases of consumption to stop the expectoration of blood.

Creosote will do this, and may suppress the cough, as well as the accompanying pain; but will it cure consumption or destroy or remove the cause of this deadliest of diseases?

On the contrary, it inevitably produces laryngeal phthisis after a very short time. It destroys the head of the windpipe and the patient dies in consequence of the destruction of one of the most important organs of the body.

In most instances the physician is either oblivious or unaware of these facts. He follows those old-standing doctrinal sophisms laid down by human "science" but discredited by nature.

His courage is called "audacity" by those who have not lost all feeling for humanity.

Meanwhile, those who regard medical science from a business standpoint only, are very quick to pronounce judgement upon any natural treatment of disease and to condemn the most successful natural physicians as charlatans and frauds.

In order to be competent to decide upon a correct course in the treatment of disease the physician must possess a thorough chemical knowledge of all the fundamental substances of which the human organism is constructed. With the patient therefore rests the responsibility of choosing his physician, since no physician can be of any assistance who cannot define what substances are deficient in the blood, and who does not possess the requisite technical knowledge to supply this deficiency by adequate dietetic means.

In my nutrition cell-food therapy for constitutional diseases, I have followed consistently upon the lines of one of the greatest masters of physiological chemistry that the world has known, who, in one of his medical colloquies spoke as follows: "In order to thoroughly understand any form of sickness or disease, so as to undertake the cure of the same, it is first of all necessary to picture before one's mental vision the ways and means of its inceptive formation, and by degrees to trace its origin, step by step, before one is enabled to decide upon adequate remedial measures conformable to the individual stages of the same."

In this sense it has ever been my strenuous endeavor to fathom the secret of the inception of constitutional diseases; but the entire medical literature did not advance me further than pathological anatomy, which informs us that the original cause of disease is a change in the form of the cellular elements of different digestive organs,—in explanation of which the customary technical terms are used, such as "atrophy," "degeneration," "metamorphosis," etc. But, I reasoned with myself, this surely cannot be seriously regarded as the origin of disease!

The cause of the visible changing of the cellules must be sought in the conditional interstitial substances which cause the invisible changes or shiftings of the cellular forms, and which are scientifically termed "*Changed nutritional conditions.*"

By the aid of physiological chemistry I was successful in finding a pathway to the centre of those mysterious occurrences of life.

And this was my course of reasoning: As the cellules, which are the smallest individual elements of the human system, are only *products of the blood*, and for their composition require the different chemical substances in sufficient quantities, it is obviously necessary to fathom what those chemical elements of the cellules may be, what form they take in their mutual relation to the separate parts of the body, and in what way they enter the organism.

In this manner I obtained a clear insight into the actions of the so-called *mineral material* in the organism, and it gradually became obvious to me that everything is dependent upon the introduction of the proper *sanguifying or nutritive* mineral salts into the blood.

On this basis I founded the so-called "*organic nutritive cell-food therapy*" (called the Dech-Manna therapy).

The point may be raised that the elements of the food we eat or drink are heterogeneous and that the mineral matter in them is naturally and casually acquired, according to the properties of the soil they grow in. This is the general opinion, but not the fact. Our vegetables, grain, meat and milk contain too much phosphoric acid and sal ammoniac, and this is due to the use of artificial and animal fertilizers, while the sulphurics are very often entirely missing.

Von Liebig says: When we consider that the sugar refineries of Waghausel have an annual output in the market of 600,000 lbs. of potassic salt, which is taken from the soil by the turnips of the Baden fields without being replaced, and that there is cultivated in Northern Germany, year by year, with the assistance of guano, an immense amount of potatoes solely for the manufacture of spirits, and that these potato fields are consequently robbed of the essential ingredients which potatoes should contain, and as these elements are only partially replaced by the insufficient component parts of the guano, we cannot be in doubt as to the condition of these fields. The ground may be ever so rich in ingredients, but it is exhaustible. The analysis of our blood indicates that, in order to remain healthy, it must contain twice as many sulphuric as phosphoric salts.

We talk glibly about a natural mode of living, a simple diet; but where in our civilized countries can we find food that really serves healthy sanguification?

The crux of the question is this: Why do we propose to *heal naturally* and not also to *nourish naturally*? — The latter is, to say the least of it, just as important as the former. But if both were practiced conjointly, a beneficial object might be more quickly and surely gained.

It is true, we are taught to eat more vegetables than meat; that our bread lacks the chief nourishing qualities, and so on; but we have hitherto been in no wise informed as to the substances that are relatively harmful or beneficial to us.

Why is it then that the science of the sanative power of nature, as well as medical science, is still in doubt in regard to the relation that must absolutely exist between the separate component parts of our nourishment in order to obtain normal healthy sanguification?

The reason is that the application of a real chemistry of life has never been comprehended until now.

According to my judgment it is Von Liebig and Julius Hensel who showed us the paths we are to take to the field of enquiry most important of all; for without a sound body all the coveted acquisitions of modern times are worthless to us.

The solution of the question how to prevent the degeneration of mankind would be a simple and natural one, if history and proverb had not taught us that as often as a new truth appears "the very oxen butt their horns against it." They cannot help this, the "disposition" is natural; for when Pythagoras had found the Master of Arts, Mathesios, he was so overjoyed that he sacrificed one hundred oxen to the gods, and ever since that time oxen are attacked with an hereditary fright whenever a new truth appears, — the human ox is no exception.

Of what use to us, for instance, are the Roentgen X-rays in diseases of the nerves when there is a generally diseased condition of the blood, which, as we now know, is also the primary cause of lung, liver, stomach and kidney troubles, cancer, scrofula, rheumatism, gout, obesity, diabetes, and the rest?

In such cases *chemistry* is necessary, in order to ascertain what ingredients are missing in the blood; they cannot be detected microscopically.

What blunders are continually committed in the treatment of nerve diseases! No one considers the physiological law that *no parts of the nerves can perform their functions lastingly and naturally unless they are continually supplied with blood permeated* with oxygen; and for this purpose iron is most necessary as an adequate ingredient.

Physicians of the old-school do prescribe iron plentifully, but in inorganic form; and because it is not organized it is indigestible and is excreted. That is why the treatment of the diseases of the nerves, which are so general and widespread, has been so unsuccessful.

It is not generally known that organized ammonium phosphate (Lecithin), which is the mineral foundation of the Neurogen I prescribe, will regenerate the nerve cells if consumed in the proper proportions. It is, likewise, little known that although a person with diseased lungs be placed under conditions where he may acquire an ample quantity of pure air—that is oxygen—and may consume as much as four quarts of milk daily, he will nevertheless most certainly be doomed to perish if his food does not contain the elements of iron, lime and sulphur in sufficient quantities.

These simple physiological laws have been ignored and medical men have given us instead, the teachings of the school of bacteriology with its pitiful illusions and its endless train of suffering and sorrow.

The testimony of many patients who have undergone treatment in the best physical culture and so-called, natural healing establishments both in Europe and America, serves to show that their success has been but partial and one-sided; that is, they have abandoned their wrong albumen theory, and their state of health has consequently improved. But, practically, the treatment has failed; for complete and final recovery—that is, full and correct nutrition and strengthening of the nerves, has not been accomplished. Such failure is due to the fact that certain essential constituents have not been supplied. These vital constituents my organic nutritive cell-food therapy is designed to provide.

What is lacking in the field of practical science, as authoritatively voiced by the unprogressive faculty of today, is an absence of chemical knowledge, especially on the part of the physician and the naturalist; and, as likewise, the so-called scientific farmer upon whose assurances we so naturally rely for the wholesome production of food is woefully ignorant on matters of agricultural chemistry, the logical consequence is that in all civilized countries great mistakes have been unconsciously made and perpetuated, detrimental to the health of man and beast alike and vitally prejudicial to the healthy sustenance of the race.

Where are the most vitally necessary mineral substances to be found in nature?

It is an established fact that the fields, on which our nutritive salts or cell-foods—our vital sustenance—are grown, were originally formed from decayed primitive rock and *this primitive earth-crust matter is composed of the same mineral substances that are found in normal blood*. Therefore, our physical welfare and our capacity to resist disease is clearly dependent upon the condition of our fields. We must always bear this in mind—the old truism—that,

"AS A MAN EATS, SO IS HE."

We are thus, directly, the products of our fields.

Wrongly fertilized, our fields must produce sickly vegetation, and this in turn will produce a sickly race and disease in cattle.

Primitive rock consists of granite, porphyry, gneiss and basalt, deposits which are still found upon the earth in immense quantities, and in the same condition as thousands of years ago.

As a matter of fact, proposals have been made by noted scientists to utilize pulverized rock of this kind as compost to *assist* the fields in a natural way, and so to restore them to their former producing power, which would thus enable plants, animals, and man, alike, to regain those substances indispensable to proper sanguification and general growth.

The agricultural experiments performed with this stone dust fully confirm this assumption.

One of the most important tasks of today is to indicate to the farmer new ways and means of promoting and increasing growth for the food supply of the nations.

Why, then, I imagine I can hear it asked, if this fact be true and demonstrated, has it not been applied?

This question may be answered by another. Why does not the natural system of Hygienic Dietetic Healing find general application in cases of sickness, since its success is so obviously greater than even that claimed by medical science?

To this vital question upon which so much of human life and happiness depends, the weak and degrading answer must suffice; to the effect that the last vestige of public respect for the sciences would be shaken, and many wise theories would fail of their imaginary virtues and succumb, before humanity's best birthright—the quality of healthy blood, kind nature's ample gift to all,—could be wrested from the selfish hand of tyranny and mankind enabled to secure from nature's willing hand the succour that an Infinite Providence offers to disease.

A physician to whom I once explained my theories, heard me for some minutes and then he said "Well, and so you want to create healthy blood in this way?" "Yes, surely," I replied. "We have no use for that," he callously exclaimed, "there would *be no business in that.*"

Hence Mankind must degenerate and Disease of all kinds ride rampant through the land, rather than upset the firmly rooted fallacies of the past or foil the ghoul-like greed of a certain set of conscienceless practitioners.

To the first of these the terse old Latin satire would apply:

"Homine imperito nunquam quidquam injustius
Qui, nisi quod ipse fecit, nihil rectum putat."

(Terentius.)

"Who is there so unreasoning as he, that learned drone,
Who reckons nothing perfect save what he himself hath known."

(M.B.)

To the second let an outraged public reply.

But meanwhile, as the hideous holocaust proceeds, the mills of God grind slowly but mysteriously secure. The eternal law of equity is working still; and from every evil there proceeds a good. Truth may be hidden in the nether deeps, but some day the strained tension breaks, the balance reversing brings it to the light. Its spirit works for ever, like a ferment, hidden long, deep down in the Universal heart of things; for with majestic, unimpressionable tread, sublimely the silent force of human progress moves; slow and inevitably sure, the great indwelling spirit of a vast eternal energy leading man ever upward to the True and Best.

Against this axiom, alas, graceless and suicidal seems the unwisdom of the world, in action against all who offer it salvation from its pain; aye, though he be Christ or Commoner.

Rather be wrong in league with wealth and power than be right—and stand alone. This is now the worldly wisdom of the sage.

Genius at grips with material and religious power, fares ill; as with far-famed Copernicus, or "starry Galileo and his woes"; or, in a brave woman's daring words:—"He, who dares to see a truth not recognized in creeds, must die the death."

"A time of transition is a time of pain," is a truism well recognized by all, and he who would press Regeneration upon the world—weak, weary and unthinking as its people are—must run the gauntlet of the bitter antagonism of the exploiting clans on this benighted sphere, though later he may see, across the bourne that bounds life's earthly day, a stately monument, perchance, by gratitude upreared, where pious crowds pay tribute to his name.

HYMN OF HEALTH

(From the Greek)

Health, thou most frangible of heaven's dower,
With thee may what remains of life be spent;
Cease not upon me, thus, thy gifts to shower,
And in my soul to find a tenement.

For what is there of beauty, wealth or power,
Of gentle offspring, or the wiles of love,
But owes its solace, sweet, in every hour,
To thee, thou regent of the powers above.

The spring of pleasure blooms if thou but bless,
And every step upon the Autumn way
Is lit by thee, parent of happiness!
Without thee sadly sounds life's roundelay.

(M.B.)

Health is one of those intangible inestimably precious posses-
sions, like life and liberty, to which all are entitled by natural Law.
Yet are there but few who are careful to conserve this priceless heritage. It is a boon all too often unappreciated until lost, and once
lost, it may not always be regained, though intense be our regrets
and our endeavours exhaust the field of human resource.

Again, although the possession of passable health may be ours, it
is a condition rarely totally untroubled and continuous and, therefore, cannot be correctly classified as perfect health.

These simple definitions may seem to the reader trite and trivial;
but how many of us, let me ask, give thought to their vital vast significance.

Never to need a physician; ever to be unconsciously guarded
against all access of disease; to maintain the fair form and vigor of

the body without effort, so that no depleting influences can find a hold; this is the health ideal by nature set, the standard to which the earliest progenitors of our race may doubtless have conformed, but upon which succeeding generations have sedulously turned their backs.

Philosophers have defined this physically perfect state.

Historians have immortalized it in heroic tomes.

Poets have extolled it in great epic verse.

Artists have depicted it in portraiture and tapestry.

Sculptors have expressed it in the life-like stone.

The sick have longed for it.

Saints have prayed for it and, in the search for its fabled, false elixir, alchemists have sacrificed their lives. It remained for the smug, "sober judgment" of our day to pronounce it "unattainable" — unattainable!

This, however, is a matter of small moment; for, as Whittier reminds us: "The falsehoods which we spurn today were the truths of long ago" — and although men part reluctantly with favorite — and lucrative — fallacies, and "Faith, fantastic Faith, once wedded fast to some dear falsehood, hugs it to the last," nevertheless this false belief, like so many other sapient pronouncements of human wisdom, must be subjected to final reversal.

The ideal state of health is, truly, "unattainable" when we refuse to yield obedience to the simple laws of nature — when we continuously persist in interference with her work and embarrass her with artificial substitutes, defying her august hygienic precepts by our manner of life.

Not so, however, if we yield to her inducements, fulfil her requirements, and submit ourselves freely to her unerring will.

There is less of fault than of weakness in the fact that so many of us fail to give nature the opportunity to rear us as healthy men and women, to keep us more free than we are from suffering and disease.

Her ways are ways of pleasantness and follow on the lines of the veriest simplicity.

The preservation of health must needs, then, move along these self-same simple lines.

It is ignorance, in most cases, rather than unwillingness that brings upon the race the punishment we call disease.

But how can they be expected to learn who have no teacher? And how can they teach who are themselves untaught?

It is incumbent upon those who have acquired knowledge to impart life-saving truths, and *there is no greater benefactor of his kind than he who reduces life's problems to their simplest terms.*

"He that dwelleth in the secret place of the Most High shall abide under the shadow of the Almighty." Such is the dictum of King David, the psalmist, as expressed in the Hebrew Scriptures.

All that man's intellect can conceive of the Almighty is bounded by its expression in Nature.

It is neither arrogant, nor irreverent, then, to claim with reasonable confidence that the devoted service of long years of close application to research in Nature's secret dwelling-place may entitle such an one to share the guidance of the Almighty mind and inspire him to share its favours with his fellow man.

This then, the Author of this brochure, realizing vividly and with sympathy, humanity's sore need, has been constrained to formulate, for the benefit of those desirous to learn;—a means of enlightenment suitable and accessible to all. For although, to quote from Goethe, whose transcendent mind was almost omniscient in all mundane things:

"Allwissend bin ich nicht; doch viel ist mir bewusst."
(Omniscient am I not, though much I know.)

Yet "Unity is strength," and in conjunction with associated minds, such knowledge as I have may amply suffice to save many a sad sufferer from hereditary doom.

The scheme, or, to be more explicit, the Club, I purpose to inaugurate, is fully expounded in detail in the succeeding pages.

THE DARE TO BE HEALTHY CLUB

All other things the mandate, "must", obey,
Man only has the power, "I will", to say.

(After Schiller.)

(M.B.)

Thoughtless and imitative, men follow custom, careless where it may lead, and unconsciously imitate each other.

Strong harmful habits grow, which overcome the opposing will and fickle fashion rules where common sense should reign.

Such instances are common to us all.

A combination opposed to such influences is the force we need and for this purpose I propose to establish a Club for the study of the ways and means of health.

THE DARE TO BE HEALTHY CLUB.

The Club will be comprised of those who desire to pursue a course of Health Study by correspondence.

This combination will constitute the first and only Club of its kind in the world.

It will unite in its membership a group of independent thinkers, representative of all parts of the American Continent.

The purpose of the Club will be to teach the science of Regeneration—to teach them to "dare to be healthy" according to the laws and teachings of biology.

These teachings will consist of a two years' course in *Biology*, dealing with its most important branches, in *Physiology*, *Anatomy*, *Hygiene*, *Physiological Chemistry*, *Pathology*, according to biological facts, and *Therapy* in accordance with biological and physical laws and precepts.

All methods of *natural healing* will be explained in detail, including diet, breathing exercises, and rest.

The comprehensive aim will be to inculcate the principles which govern the process of perfect metabolism — that is to say, the changes of nutritive matter within the body — as the means of bringing into being a race endowed with health and beauty and therefore predestined to happiness.

The course of instruction will be based upon the literature of science, including certain fundamental teachings from the pen of the author of the present pamphlet, which comprises, moreover, extracts from the works of distinguished scholars whose theories have been tried and tested during the last thirty-five years.

Its precepts will be based upon personal experience and actual practice, the outcome of careful and patient observation.

The series throughout will be formulated with a view to the purpose of graduating later from among those who follow the course, a body of competent instructors capable of transmitting the knowledge they have acquired to others, privately or professionally. But remember the axiom of Cicero:

"Not only is there an art in acquiring knowledge but also a rarer art in imparting it to others."

The first question, then, which will naturally arise in the mind of the reader will be:

What is This Method of Regeneration?

The reply to this question is in reality a simple one, but in order to explain and define the word "Regeneration" from a purely scientific standpoint, it will be necessary to cite the results of the author's researches and to outline his method of healing by regeneration, showing how he purposes to lead the way from a dark past and a dull present into a brighter future.

Before doing so, however, it may perhaps conduce to a better understanding if I quote from the remarks of an eminent local authority on the chemical composition of the body — a subject "new," as it appears, to the general medical practitioner of the day though, for over a quarter of a century freely expatiated upon by the great Biologists of the period.

The extract is taken from a recent article by Assistant Surgeon General Dr. W.C. Rucker, of the United States Public Health Service, and reads as follows:

"Much of the advance of modern medicine has been accomplished through the development of physiological chemistry which is even yet a new science.

"Although so new, it is assuming such importance as to make it manifest that the physiology of the future will be written largely in terms of chemistry.

"We have come to realize that the body is in a literal sense of the word, a chemical laboratory. The foods we eat, the fluids we drink, the gases we breathe are complex chemical compounds which the body must take apart and put together again in such a way that the materials may be delivered in a shape that will enable the cells to store them. It is then the business of the cells to utilize these materials for TISSUE BUILDING and in the production of energy, in the form of work and heat. The body manufactures different kinds of products, some beneficial, others harmful. Thus for example, excessive muscular effort throws into the bloodstream fatigue products that are poisonous. A person utterly tired out is really suffering from acute poisoning. On the other hand, to resist invasion by infectious diseases, the body manufactures anti-poisons that kill the enemy germs — making in other words, its own medicine."

The physical processes here mentioned by Dr. Rucker are fully explained in my book, "Dare to be Healthy," chapter VI, VII, VIII, and the natural principles involved have been practiced by me for over 30 years. I mention the fact simply as corroborative evidence of the authenticity and value of the work shortly to be published.

"Art may err, but Nature cannot miss," — is an aphorism attributed to the poet Dryden. It adequately supports Dr. Rucker's wise, significant and timely pronouncement and reminds me of an illustrative incident recorded in connection with the world famed physician Boerhaave of Leyden, — Holland's chief centre of learning —

who lived some 250 years ago, when doctors knew less than at present of the circulation and functions of the blood.

Boerhaave, it appears, conceived the idea of a sort of posthumous pleasantry, of a distinctly lucrative nature, at the expense of his medical brethren. Professional ignorance and popular superstition had alike surrounded his name with a halo of mystery and he was credited with almost miraculous powers of healing and the possession of the Secret of Disease and Health.

At the sale of effects, following his death, there was a great gathering of the most celebrated physicians of the day and his books and records fetched fabulous prices. But one special tome, ponderous, silver-clasped and locked, entitled: "Macrobiotic, The True and Complete Secret of Long, Healthy Life," was the cynosure of every avaricious eye. The auctioneer shrewdly reserved it until the last. Amidst a scene of unparalleled excitement and competition the Great Book was at length knocked down to a famous London physician for no less a sum than seven thousand Gulden. When opened with eager anticipation before the disappointed bidders, its pages were found to be blank—with one exception. Upon this one was inscribed in the handwriting of Boerhaave himself, only these ten words:

"Keep the head cool, the feet warm, the bowels open."

Turning to an excited audience it was thus the great London authority spoke:

"I once heard it said that the world is simple; that health is simple; that it is the folly of man that causes all complications, and that it is the delicate task of the true physician to reduce everything to its original simplicity. Heaven knows that our great Master, Boerhaave, has solved life's problem. To me this truth is well worth the 7,000 Gulden I pay to secure it; while to you, my friends, who have travelled from distant parts of the globe in search of it, receive from me the legacy of our Master and also be, likewise, content."

The moral that this story teaches is the same eternal lesson of all time, as expressed through the medium of Biology: that not by art or artifice can health be cheaply snatched at will from the Infinite Sources of Life, but that by consistently following the guidance of

Nature's Laws the healthy functions of the human organism may alone be correctly maintained, or, when driven by ill-treatment into decline, it is the rational scientific assistance we afford to the efforts of Nature, by which alone we may hope to re-establish that normal condition of health. For, in the worthy words of Wordsworth I may say: "So build we up the being that we are."

The writer does not claim for this method so great a degree of simplicity. But he does base it upon the same truth that simplicity and a return to natural conditions are the only ways of effectively healing the diseased body.

Guided by the great masters of biology and physiological chemistry, his object has been to determine the elements of which the twelve main tissues of the human body are composed and to learn in what manner these tissues suffer from the various diseases which attack them.

Were I desirous of emulating the illustrious Boerhaave, I might concentrate my work into these few words: *Supply the system with the necessary constituents of its tissues and at the same time assist the organism by means of simple and natural appliances, and REGENERATION will continue until the desired physiological condition is reached.*

In so doing, I fear, I should bequeath but little to the comprehension of humanity.

I desire that all shall benefit by the diligent research work of my life. I desire to leave my legacy to humankind clearly and distinctly defined, in rules carefully expressed in the Course of Study I have prepared.

I do not expect them to be accepted without controversy. Nor do I look for gratitude from those whom I seek to benefit. I have no delusions and the satisfaction of having delivered my message will be my sole reward. I can only trust in this more enlightened age, that history as poetized by Pope may not repeat itself:

> "Truths would you teach, or save a sinking land?
> All fear, none aid you, and few understand."

My solace, even so, for the nonce would be the knowledge of life and health restored to the faithful, though, comparatively, few and the confidence that truth must, in the issue, at length prevail, convincing, victorious over all.

Before proceeding further I wish it to be distinctly understood that it is no part of my scheme or intention to seek in any way to eliminate the physician.

As there are, in fact, no two human organism exactly alike, so also is there divergence, more or less, in each individual case, in disease; and however apparently similar the symptoms may be, the knowledge and experience of a physician becomes necessary in order to determine correctly what the ailment is and how general principles should be applied in each particular case.

On the contrary, I purpose to explain fully the secret causes of disease and their removal, in pursuance of the belief held in common with fair-minded physicians the world over, that a better knowledge of the human organism and hygiene on the part of the layman, would be of equal advantage alike to physician and patient.

Drawing aside the veil from professional secrecy and allowing the patient to know the why and the wherefore of things, means positive success for my hygienic-dietetic system of healing, because it is the only system which can ultimately survive in the light of general knowledge and wisdom.

No knowledge, no precautions, will always prevent disease. It is the natural incidence of the law of cause and effect that man, collectively, cannot expect to go through life unmolested by disturbances of health. From the very outset the tendency to disease is inherited; and indeed today, although we have now learned how to combat the enemy, yet opposing hosts are seen to be so vast and strongly entrenched about us that we realize to some extent the years that must elapse before mankind can be entirely set free from his hideous heritage, the harvest sown by past ignorance, deception and neglect.

But, from the malignant evil of internecine strife Universal Good is rising with an awakened nation's cry—a cry for freedom and release from the ever-lengthening chains of pernicious interests and obsolete institutions. The moment of release is at hand: That pyschological moment of which James Russell Lowell sings:

> "Once to every man and nation
> Comes the moment to decide,
> In the strife of Truth with Falsehood,
> For the good or evil side."

And knowing what the People know — they who have borne so long, in grimly impotent silence, under the guise of Freedom, the fortunes of the slave — can we for one moment doubt what view their lawful, reasoning demand for redress will take and whether or no it will prevail? The hundred million voices of the Union sternly answer: NO!

In effecting this release, so far as the Science of Healing is concerned, my system, which I claim to be entirely original, will be found particularly efficacious, for it presents plainly and convincingly, in the light of the most recent discoveries, the truth that *all constitutional diseases are but the variations of one basal deficiency*; that the entire art of rational healing lies in a knowledge of the component parts of the body tissues, in a determination of the tissues involved in the process of degeneration in each specific instance, and in the subsequent treatment thereof by means of supplying to the blood the elements necessary to regenerate the tissues in question.

From this brief explanation may be judged the importance of the hygienic dietetic physician in cases of sickness. The quack and charlatan it is who persuade people to believe that they do not need the physician, and compel them to pay for this belief in money and in health. It is the obvious duty of every one to seek aid in case of sickness from some physician who is a profound and professed advocate of the only sensible, practical method of treatment; but, at the same time I would make it possible for all to acquire sufficient knowledge to enable them to judge for themselves whether the attendant summoned responds in some measure to this requirement, the simple and logical course of which contains at least some ray of hope for all who suffer.

It may not be amiss to cite here a brief outline of the teachings of the four bright particular stars who have served as beacon lights in the history and development of medicine. Not only does the modern medical world acknowledge the doctrines of these four men as the foundation upon which the practice of healing has been raised to a science, but moreover,—*a point much more important for our consideration*,—it also admits that the least essential part of the work of Hippocrates, the "Father of Medicine;" namely, his *statement of theory*, is the part which has been accorded permanent prominence, whilst the portion of greatest value in his labours; that is to say, the *practical part*, has been neglected and ignored.

The following passages are taken from the article entitled "History of Medicine" in the Encyclopedia Britannica, 11th. Edition, vol. XVIII, pages 42-51.

"*Hippocrates*, called the 'Father of Medicine,' lived during the age of Pericles, (495-429 B.C.), and occupied as high a position in medicine as did the great philosophers, orators, and tragedians in their respective fields.

His high conception of the duties and position of the physician and the skill with which he manipulated the materials that were at hand, constituted two important characteristics of Hippocratic medicine. Another was the recognition that disease, as well as health, is a process governed by what we call natural laws, learned by observation, and indicating the direction of recovery. These views of the 'natural history of disease' led to habits of minute observation and careful interpretation of symptoms, in which the Hippocratic school excelled and has been the model for all succeeding ages, so that even now the true method of clinical medicine may be said to be the method of Hippocrates.

One of the important doctrines of Hippocrates was the healing power of nature. He did not teach that nature was sufficient to cure disease, but he recognized a natural process of the humours, at least in acute disease, being first of all *crude*, then passing through *coction* or digestion, and finally being expelled by resolution or crisis through one of the natural channels of the body. The duty of the physician was to 'assist and not to hinder these changes, so that the sick man might conquer the disease with the help of the physician.'"

"*Galen*, the man from whom the greater part of modern European medicine has flowed, lived about 131 to 201 A.D. He was equipped with all the anatomical, medical, and philosophical knowledge of his time; he had studied all kinds of natural curiosities and was in close touch with important political events; he possessed enormous industry, great practical sagacity, and unbounded literary fluency. At that time there were numerous sects in the medical profession, various dogmatic systems prevailed in medical science, and the social standing of physicians was degraded. He assumed the task of reforming the existing evils and restoring the unity of medicine as it had been understood by Hippocrates, at the same time elevating the dignity of medical practitioners.

In the explanation and healing of diseases he applied the science of physiology. His theory was based upon the Hippocratic doctrine of humours, but he developed it with marvelous ingenuity. He advocated that the normal condition of the body depended upon a proper proportion of the four elements, hot, cold, wet and dry. The faulty proportions of the same gave rise, not to disease, but to the occasions for disease. He laid equal stress upon the faulty composition or dysaemia of the blood. He claimed that all diseases were due to a combination of these morbid predispositions, together with injurious external influences, and thus explained all symptoms and all diseases. He found a name for every phenomenon and a solution for every problem. And though it was precisely in this characteristic that he abandoned scientific methods and practical utility, it was also this quality that gained for him his popularity and prominence in the medical world.

However, his reputation grew slowly. His opinions were in opposition to those of other physicians of his time. In the succeeding generation he won esteem as a philosopher, and it was only gradually that his system was accepted implicitly. It enjoyed great, though not exclusive predominance until the fall of Roman civilization."

" *Thomas Sydenham*, (1624-1689) was well acquainted with the works of the ancient physicians and had a fair knowledge of chemistry. Whether he had any knowledge of anatomy is not definitely known. He advocated the actual study of disease in an impartial manner, discarding all hypothesis. He repeatedly referred to Hippocrates in his medical methods, and he has quite deservedly been styled the English Hippocrates. He placed great stress on the 'natural history of disease,' just as did his Greek master, and likewise attached great importance to 'epidemic constitution,' that is, the influence of weather and other natural causes on the process of disease. He believed in the healing power of nature to an even greater degree than did Hippocrates. He claimed that disease was nothing more than an effort on the part of nature to restore the health of the patient by the elimination of the morbific matter.

The reform of practical medicine was effected by men who advocated the rejection of all hypothesis and the impartial study of natural processes, as shown in health and disease. Sydenham showed that these natural processes could be studied and dealt with without being explained, and, by laying stress on facts and disregarding *explanations*, he introduced a *method* in medicine far more fruitful than any discoveries. Though the dogmatic spirit continued to live for a long time, the reign of standard authority had passed."

"*Boerhaave.* In the latter part of the seventeenth century a physician arose (1668-1738) who was destined to become far more prominent in the medical world than any of the English physicians of the age of Queen Anne, though he differed but little from them in his way of thinking. This was *Hermann Boerhaave*. For many years he was professor of medicine at Leyden, and excelled in influence and reputation not only his greatest forerunners, Montanus of Padua and Sylvius of Leyden, but probably every subsequent teacher. The Hospital of Leyden became the centre of medical influence in Europe. Many of the leading English physicians of the 18th century studied there. Boerhaave's method of teaching was transplanted to Vienna through one of his pupils, Gerard Van Swieten, and thus the noted Vienna school of medicine was founded.

The services of Boerhaave to the progress of medicine can hardly be overestimated. He was the organizer and almost the constructor of the modern method of clinical instruction. He followed the methods of Hippocrates and Sydenham in his teachings and in his practice. The points of his system that are best known are his doctrines of inflammation, obstruction, and 'plethora.' In the practice of medicine he aimed to make use of all the anatomical and physiological acquisitions of his age, including microscopical anatomy.

In this respect he differed from Sydenham, for the latter paid but little more attention to modern medicine than to ancient dogma. In some respects he was like Galen, but again differed from him, as he did not wish to reduce his knowledge to any definite system. He spent much time in studying the medical classics, though he valued them from an historical standpoint rather than from an authoritative standpoint. It would almost seem that the great task of Boerhaave's life a combination of ancient and modern medicine, could not be of any real permanent value, and the same might be said of his Aphorisms, in which he gave a summary of the results of his long experience. And yet it is an indisputable fact that his contributions to the science of medicine form one of the necessary factors in the construction of modern medicine."

These extracts represent the principles of that bright constellation of Master Minds who have gone before us and guided our footsteps through tedious and tentative wanderings into the pathway of Truth. May their undoubting, united testimony act as a reassuring, convincing influence which will carry the reader back to the very fountain head of Medical jurisprudence, through the medium of the Encyclopedia Britannica, the highest accepted authority and criterion of authenticity in the English speaking world; for, at the same time it will also provide a positive and perfect safeguard and assurance of the solid basis and absolute authenticity of my methods and teachings besides indicating definitely the source and direction whence they are derived and establishing their classical trend and legitimate purpose.

SYSTEM OF REGENERATION

In order to bring the entire system of regeneration under review, I shall here endeavour to present in condensed form all the essential points in my teachings. The reader will thus be enabled to picture to himself his body, with its vital organs, clearly as in a mirror; he will become familiarized with its composition and twelve principal tissues, as well as with the sixteen elements of which they consist.

Man is a unit, and the human body an accumulation of millions of separate cells, which are centres of life and which, in different groupings and combinations, form the various organs that render existence possible.

This existence is the natural sequel of the existence of former human beings. They generated the life that is to be transferred by us to other living beings.

The several functions of the organism combine to form a chain of activities in which there must not be a single link missing, if life is to continue.

These activities are comprised within an accumulation of cells which are by no means stationary, for life means nothing more than the constant dying, of the old cells and the reconstruction of the new. It means that the human body as a whole is continually in a state of composition and decomposition.

Not until the accumulation of cells we call the body is recognized as one complete correlated and inseparable entity and the absolute interdependence of the separate cells, each one upon the others, is likewise accepted as the verified fact that it is—not until then will the erroneous and obsolete idea be discarded, by which the various organs of the body have been professionally treated as separate and independent considerations, even to the extent of being dealt with, in cases of disease, as totally aloof from one another and conveniently classed as proper subjects for submission to the expert opinion of that superior class of physicians who devote their attention exclusively to special organs and are accordingly termed "Specialists."

Thus the question arises: What is the cause of *disease*? The question does not apply to any one particular form of disease or class of diseases, but to disease generally, as a concrete term meaning any disorder which may manifest itself by individual disturbances in the body; for such disturbance is but a variation in quantity or quality of one general disturbance, a variation in the mechanism that controls the work of keeping the existing cells in proper condition and replacing those cells which are constantly being destroyed. It is a variation in the process of *regeneration, which we term life.*

METABOLISM is the process which is constantly going on in the human system, whereby the cells that have been consumed by oxidation are removed through the excreta — the faeces, the urine, the perspiration, and the exhalations from the lungs — to be replaced by new ones.

Metabolism, means change of matter. It signifies the course by which nutritive material, or food, is built up into living matter. This process is accomplished through the blood, which distributes the necessary material to all parts of the body where cells need to be replaced and carries away the consumed portions.

In the marvelous performance of its functions, when properly supplied, it carries the elements that are essential to regeneration in the correct proportions. When not properly supplied, these proportions become incorrect and foreign formations may arise which are disturbing to the organism.

In nature there is a constant tendency to counterbalance disturbances in the proper proportion and by distribution of cell building material to restore the normal condition. We may thus speak of the overwhelmingly curative tendency of nature.

Metabolism is the function of the body which most constantly requires attention. So, therefore, it is always through the blood that we must assist nature in the process of counterbalancing and rectifying or healing abnormal conditions.

It follows then, that, despite the apparent variety in *constitutional* diseases, they are all practically the same. They are all disturbances of metabolism through some irregularity in the quantitative or qualitative condition of the blood.

Professor Jacob Moleschott, the great physiologist, has crystallized this truth in the immortal words: "One of the principal questions to be always asked of the physician is this: How may good healthy and active blood be obtained? View the question as we may, we shall be forced to acknowledge openly and explicitly or guardedly and indirectly that our volition, our sensations, our strength, and our pro-creative powers are dependent upon our blood and our blood upon our nutrition."

If such unity exists, why then the great difference in the human organs? How is it that a bone in its stonelike hardness is essentially the same as the exquisitely sensitive eye?

This is owing to the adaptive property of the cells, in the course of their enormous accumulation, to different functions, which, again, depends upon the varied arrangement of the constituent elements. These elements all find lodgement in the blood, and are carried by it in necessary quantities to the points where they are needed to assist the organs in replacing consumed matter.

The difficulty found in grasping this idea of *unity* has led to the most momentous errors in modern medical science.

One result has been the undue attention paid to the study of anatomy, insomuch that the different organs are regarded as wholly distinct groups of cells. This is convenient from a descriptive stand-point, but it tends too much to draw attention away from the source of life, and of health. Only by noting the common characteristics of the cell accumulations termed organs, are we enabled to supply the necessary elements that may be lacking. And thus we arrive at the subject of *the chemical analysis of the human body* and its various organs, a subject that has been badly neglected throughout the centuries.

It has been determined that the entire human body consists of a certain number of chemical elements, appearing in different aggregations in different parts. These aggregations repeating themselves in the various organs.

Twelve principal aggregations of chemical elements have been established and designated by the term *tissues.*

This fact led to the discovery of the truth that in the process of healing attention must be given, not to the various organs, but to the various tissues.

These tissues are dependent directly upon the condition and contents of the blood, whose office it is to nourish them and which exhibits the wonderful property of conveying to each tissue its selective regenerative materials, *provided of course, that these elements are present at the time in the blood.*

Sixteen definite elements have been established—and a seventeenth will probably soon be added thereto—which, in their various combinations and aggregations, form the different tissues of which the organs in the human body are composed.

The prevalence of one or several of these elements in a certain tissue forms the main or governing feature of that tissue. Thus, the prevalence of potassium phosphate characterizes muscle tissue, the prevalence of ammonium phosphate (lecithin) nerve tissue. Each one of the various tissues consists of certain of these elements, and each tissue at every point where it occurs is affected by the lack of any of its elements.

One of the greatest physiological chemists, Justus von Liebig, maintains that, if one of the necessary elements in a chemical composition is missing, the rest cannot fulfill their duties and the respective cells must become diseased and degenerate.

This discovery, known as "the law of the minimum," has thrown additional light upon the tasks before the new school of medicine.

Upon the basis of a careful diagnosis, the necessary nutritive salts or cell-foods, carefully compounded in accordance with the law of chemotaxis must be administered. This law discovered by *Engelmann*, requires that these cell-foods must be administered in digestible and assimilable forms so that the cells will be attracted by the chemical reaction, which may be of a positive or a negative character.

This being so, we can easily build up the tissues, by studying their chemical composition and supplying to the system that which is necessary, in the form of food. The cell will take care of the rest. Each tissue has its specific cell-system, and each cell will be attracted only by those ingredients which are needed for the mother tissue.

To bring to a tissue through the blood the lacking constituent element or elements is the only means of regenerating and healing diseased cells.

In this connection we are considering only constitutional diseases.

It has been shown that the lack of certain chemical elements from the blood signifies disease and that the variety of the disease depends on which of the elements are either lacking entirely or are present in incorrect proportion.

After this lack has been determined, the course to pursue in curing the disease is to supply the lacking chemical elements in the form of concentrated cell-food in *addition* to the regular food.

This method displaces entirely the old system of filling the body with poisonous drugs in order to *counteract the effects of the disease.* Such a system may suppress the symptoms by benumbing the nerves and preventing pain, it may counteract the natural process of healing of which inflammation, fever and pain, are the outward manifestations;—*but it can never cure.*

The discovery of dysaemia, or impaired blood supply, as the governing cause of disease, has destroyed another idol of modern fetish worship in medicine.

Since the discovery of various species of bacilli, which accompany nearly every form of disease in some form or other, these have been commonly declared to be the causes of diseases, and the tendency is to find some poison that will kill the bacilli in order to cure the disease.

The bacillus, on the contrary, is only the consequence, or symptom, of a disease. The diseased and decomposing parts furnish fertile soil suitable to the propagating of bacilli because of the lack of the normal chemical elements in the blood and tissue. But to kill them, while the underlying conditions for their reproduction remain unchanged, can, obviously, never effect a cure. So the great hopes that have attached to sero-therapy are doomed to disappointment, and the application of anti-toxins prepared from the serum of animals, are fated shortly to vanish in the wake of others of those strange temporary crazes which periodically obsess mankind for a while and pass away.

The discovery that a dysaemic condition of the blood leads to certain destructive processes termed diseases, was soon followed by the apprehension that one of the principal factors in bringing about such disturbance is *predisposition,*—in many cases heredity.

The term "Hereditary disease" signifies that the improper chemical composition of the blood of one or both parents is transmitted to the offspring, and that it causes in them likewise a degeneration of certain tissues and of the organs composed of those tissues.

The hygienic-dietetic system of healing does not, however, regard heredity as an invincible enemy, especially since my discovery of the "Law of the Cross-Transmission of Characteristics."

It is in the solution of this problem of "hereditary disease" that my system will eventually come into its own and will ere long be recognized as the most rational and effectual therapy ever applied since the beginning of the art of healing. It may be years before it is accorded the proverbially tardy acknowledgment of the "orthodox" schools, but that it will, nay *must* be eventually adopted is virtually a foregone conclusion—that is, if it be indeed the function or policy of the physician of the future to adequately seek to succour the suffering and regenerate the races of mankind. Of the physician of the present it can at best be said in Goethe's incisive words:

> "Er halt die Theile in seiner Hand,
> Doch fehlt ihm leider das gelst' ge Band."

> He holds the parts within his hand,
> But lacks the mental grasp of all.

For full explanation of the significance of my law, I must refer you to the first lecture in my book entitled "Within the Bud,"—and the lesson therein on the theory of "Pangenesis," which space forbids my repeating here. This lesson will convey conclusively to any thinking mind what heredity really means. After a brief study of this interesting subject the importance of the "Law of the Cross-Transmission of Characteristics" will become amply apparent and the intelligent reader will undoubtedly wonder why it has not been applied and acknowledged long ago. For answer, I must refer you to the schools, whose policy it has ever been to, at any rate, abstain from assisting, if not absolutely to diplomatically hinder the development of fresh scientific discoveries. But the time is fast approaching when a sharp and decisive end to this iniquity will be demanded by the will of an enlightened people; only then will the existing orthodox power be compelled to loosen its obstructive grip which the interests of humanity have, so far, been powerless to unclasp. But, to quote the stirring words of one who looked with prophetic, faithful eye into the tangled problems of futurity:

"The people will come into their own at last, —
God is not mocked for ever."

My Law of the Cross-Transmission of Characteristics may be simply stated as follows:

Under all conditions, the matter of sex is determined in the egg-cell at the moment of fertilization.

Under all conditions, the sex is determined by a struggle for the mastery in the egg-cell, between the energy of that egg-cell and the energy of the male spermatozoon. In a crisis, when the life of one of the two seeds is trembling in the balance, one of them — through the exertion of its "Latent Reserve Energy," dominates, and engenders a child of the opposite sex. This reversal of the sex is in conformity with the Law of the *Cross-Transmission of Sex*; that is, the mother is represented in the male offspring and the father in the female, — this being the normal expression of the Law of Cross-Transmission of Characteristics.

The "Latent Reserve Energy" is provided by nature for the "Preservation of Species," and through this provision an impulsive, vehement energy can, at the final moment of a crisis, be called upon for the salvation of its kind.

A *seeming* exception to this is due to the "Law of the Dominant" which overrides the action of "Latent Reserve Energy," and is a provision of nature for the preservation of the "Dominant," which is the most prominent quality in nature.

When the subject is properly understood, this *seeming* exception will also become clear.

In the natural course, the study of heredity leads to the understanding of *predisposition*. In other words, if you have understood heredity, it will be easy to understand predisposition; for it means that the protoplasm or seed, from whichever organism it may proceed, must contain some of the salient characteristics of its ancestors, good and bad, dominant and recessive. Not only will it contain characteristics from father and mother, but from *all* the direct ancestors. It is impossible to know exactly which points will manifest themselves, but a good many *bad* points *may be* eliminated by studying the ancestral line; and the direct diseases or bad characteristics of a parent, *must be* eliminated by applying the Law of the Cross-Transmission of Characteristics.

For example: If the father has a certain disease or positive symptoms of that disease, by no means create a girl, as she will certainly be predisposed for that disease, and may pay the penalty, if "Regeneration" is not begun early. The same principle applies to the mother. If she is diseased, do not create a son, until "Regeneration" has been brought about.

Furthermore, it will be possible to improve the offspring by encouraging and promoting the good points, especially after studying and applying the above law, as well as my law of the "Determination of the Sex at Will."

Looking at the question from this point of view, we begin to realize the enormous significance of my discovery. This supplies the main reason for the study of the laws, for the "*Prevention of Diseases*."

Only when we know that every acquired characteristic may be transmitted to the offspring will we become conscious of the *terrible responsibility* we assume when we reproduce offspring, and realize that we may create more pain and suffering instead of eliminating it.

As Nature *demands* that we reproduce ourselves or be punished for disobeying her laws, what is to be done?

Study and follow the advice given in this book, and you will awake to the fact that Nietsche's words were not "Utopian" when he commanded us to "reproduce something better than we are."

Together with the predisposition to disease, the child also acquires the hereditary tendency to regeneration; and thus rational hygienic-dietetic treatment may be able to eliminate the diseases which were formerly pronounced incurable. This can only be effected by the effort to remove the cause and strengthen the weak points by means of Regeneration.

The reader will now plainly understand that in order to heal, according to the hygienic-dietetic system, the blood must be supplied with the chemical elements that are missing from the tissues.

There are three ways of accomplishing this; namely, by diet, by nutritive preparations, and by physical treatment.

The first and most natural way is by means of proper diet.

Since the chemical elements are introduced into the body through the food, the quantity and quality of the food must be regulated. The patient must receive food that will help in regenerating his blood; particularly such food as contains the elements that are lacking in the affected tissues in his body.

The regular supply of food is however usually insufficient to overcome the process of destruction, and it is therefore necessary to add the missing elements in purer form and larger quantity. These nutritive preparations contain only such chemical elements as exist in the human body; they also contain them in the proper chemical proportion and are entirely free from poisonous substances. They promote a general regeneration of the blood that will eventually lead to a complete cure.

Physical treatment may be made to assist the proper circulation of the blood, opening at the same time the pores of the skin for the withdrawal from the body of disease elements and the introduction of desirable material. Massage, gymnastics, ablutions, and various kinds of baths and packs constitute the most of the healing measures of this description resorted to.

This is indeed the legitimate field for Osteo-Chyropractice.

In order to understand the method of treatment which I apply, it is necessary to understand one of the great laws of physiological chemistry, acknowledged as such by the great masters of chemistry, such as Liebig and Hensel.

This law demonstrates that *nature is a unit, its component parts a given number of elements, each of which has distinct qualities, and the combination of which produces the various manifestations of life.*

These elements are classified as combining to form minerals, plants and animals. They are all closely interrelated. The plant draws the mineral elements from the soil, and after certain processes of combination, conveys them as food to the animal. The animal substances that man consumes make up the balance of the elements that are required to build up the human body.

It is a matter of comparatively new discovery that the minerals are just as important a part of the human body and of its food as the other basic chemical elements. The discovery showing of what minerals the necessary ingredients of the different body tissues are composed and in what combination and quantity, in order that they may become incorporated into the organism, has made it possible to supply them to the diseased body in the purest and most effective way through nutritive preparations, while their existence in food also furnishes an indication as to the regulation of diet.

I have already given, in the preceding pages, the frank expression of favourable opinion upon this vital topic generally, as voiced with unmistakable, conviction by no less an authority than Assistant Surgeon-General, Dr. W.C. Rucker of the United States Public Health Service. I will now cite, in further corroboration, the opinion of the distinguished Editor of "The Fra," as addressed to myself personally, in special relation to an advance section of the book "Dare to be Healthy," together with other similar matter, and which, coming as it does from one who is himself a leader in the van of the advancing phalanx of the followers of Truth and Enlightenment, may be safely held to constitute a just criterion of the literary and technical value of the work. It is expressed as follows:

From John T. Hoyle, Managing Editor of "The Fra."

"From my reading of your 'Lessons,' and especially from 'Dare to be Healthy,' I can see that you have evolved a new concept in medicine, or rather 'Nature Healing,' which promises great results. I trust you will be able to put the whole into a printed book that we may all have the benefit of your discoveries. Unlike most physicians, while you treat of the most profound and vital scientific subjects, your language is so well chosen and your method of presentation is so clear, that no intelligent person would have difficulty in following your thought. You have undertaken a monumental work, and that success may attend your efforts is our heartfelt wish."

From Elbert Hubbard.

"What I have read of it is intensely interesting and shows that you have a keen insight into the philosophies of life."

There are other spontaneous and unexpected testimonials of an equally encouraging and complimentary nature from men whose knowledge and attainments entitle their opinions to the tribute of respect. These might well be likewise added here, but for the necessary limitations of space.

When Moses saved the hosts of Israel from starvation in the desert, by obtaining the solid and liquid food requisite for their deliverance, he called the name of that food "Manna." in like manner, both as a just tribute to the success they have achieved in the past and as an earnest of the deliverance they are destined to achieve in the future, I have designated my preparations by a similar term and called them the "*Dech-Manna*" *Nutritive Preparations.*

Although presented in so condensed a form, the preceding outline cannot fail to inspire in the mind of the reader a vivid conception of the simple grandeur of nature's handiwork, more especially as regards her provisions in relation to health and disease—secrets revealed, through microscope and alembic, to those who, in spite of organized discouragement, have attempted to fathom the erstwhile mysteries of human suffering and to carry hope and freedom into the hostile camps of Fear, Disease and Death.

To bring these considerations within the comprehension of all, and to win all, so far as possible, to the practical observance of the means and precepts of Health and Safety is the object of the projected course of study of which the following is the business proposition.

THE DARE TO BE HEALTHY CLUB

BUSINESS PROPOSITION

The course of study in connection with the above consists of

A SERIES OF ONE HUNDRED LESSONS

to be issued in weekly instalments, the whole course to extend over a period of two years.

Each lesson will consist, approximately, of some twenty-two to twenty-five full-sized pages (i.e. 25/28 lines of 8/12 words each) which will be mailed to every subscriber weekly prepaid.

It is necessary, in view of contingent expenses that a membership of *One thousand subscribers* should be obtained, as only when such an amount of support is guaranteed would the printing of the hundred lectures under the easy and advantageous terms offered be at all justified.

If, however, it should be represented to me by those most immediately interested, that it is their desire to Confine the Club to narrower limits, I might, though with some reluctance, consider the advisability of reducing the minimum membership to *One hundred students* provided that these should agree to contribute the sum total of the fees for the two years course in advance.

With every twentieth lesson will be forwarded to the subscriber, gratis, one of five well bound volumes of superior literary attraction and interest.

These five volumes are as follows:

ATLAS OF HUMAN ANATOMY (profusely illustrated with coloured plates and containing folding manikin) especially compiled for the student.

MANUAL OF PHYSIOLOGY, especially compiled for the student.

MANUAL OF PHYSIOLOGICAL CHEMISTRY, especially compiled for the student.

MANUAL OF BIOLOGICAL THERAPY, Dechmann's system, (500 pages).

MEDICAL DICTIONARY (pocket edition in flexible leather with gilt edges, giving 30,000 definitions.)

At the end of the course each student in good standing, will receive free of cost a Membership Diploma in the form of a beautifully artistic colour plate, the facsimile of which will appear herewith.

"Within the Bud; the Procreation of a Healthy, Happy, and Beautiful Child of the Desired Sex, by L. Dechmann, Biologist." This is a book of 302 pages, the paper bound edition retailing at $3.00, the edition de luxe at $5.00, can be obtained at any book store or direct from the author.

The above literature cannot be otherwise procured, and its cost actually amounts to nearly one-half the subscription for the entire course of lessons.

At the close of the course a beautiful engraved cover design for binding the 100 lessons may be obtained at the price of $1.00.

Separate file binders and perforators for the lessons, each cover holding some 300 pages, may be obtained at the nominal cost of about 50 cents each; one of these will be delivered free with the first lesson.

CELL-FOODS.

In addition to these advantages, all members of the Club will be entitled to procure any supplies they may need of the Dech-Manna Cell-Foods at special (wholesale) prices.

LOUIS DECHMANN.

Biologist and Physiological Chemist.
127 North 59th Street, Seattle, Wash., U.S.A.

THE BASIS OF PROCEEDINGS

of

THE DARE TO BE HEALTHY CLUB

In the ensuing pages I shall endeavour to give the reader a necessarily brief and cursory, glance into the subjects which will form the underlying motif of the vast and manifold deliberations which will constitute the fundamental basis of the projected course of study which will be brought under the consideration of the members of the proposed association and will constitute the schedule, as it were, of the periodical dissertations of these matters of world-wide and vital individual significance to be comprised in the Series of One Hundred Lessons.

I have been at some pains to avoid as far as possible the use of technical and professional phrases and terminology, for the express purpose of bringing within the scope of every faculty of understanding these subjects which are equally *a matter of life and death importance* to every man, woman and child, in all the wide and varied range of nationalities and languages which constitute so large a part of our great Republic and upon whose health and efficiency so much of our national life depends.

The great and ominous unrest, so much in evidence of late, is ample proof of a latent popular dissatisfaction with the conditions of life and it is equally significant of the prevailing nervous tension—the obvious result of malnutrition of the system—which is one of the most prominent popular features of the worry-worn denizen of today.

Life, Health, Happiness—that vital interdependent triad—are surely a preoccupation strong enough and precious enough to startle the minds of the most complacent; and it is with the object of awakening all to their possibilities—in health or in disease—of protection of the one, and hope and regeneration under the other, that the course of study has been inaugurated of which the following is but a bare outline.

MAN AS A UNIT. [A]

The human body is an accumulation of millions of separate cells, which are the bearers of life, and which in various groups form the different organs, the combined action of which constitutes our individual existence.

This existence itself is the natural issue of the existence of our predecessors, who generated the new life which will be transmitted by us and reappear in our offspring.

In like manner all the functions of the body form an endless chain in which not a single link must be faulty or missing, if healthy organic life is to continue.

This accumulation of cells, however, is by no means inactive. On the contrary, organic life is nothing but the constant dying of the old and the reconstruction of new cells; it means that we are in a perpetual condition of composition and consequently of decomposition throughout our entire being, its different parts and organs.

As soon as we are able to recognize this accumulation of cells as one individual whole and thus arrive at the idea of their absolute interdependence, we shall get rid of the prevalent idea, that the mere structural differences between the respective organs of the body make them separate and independent things which may be treated irrespective of one another in case of disease, or dealt with by different specialists.

We arrive then at the one great question: *What is the cause of disease?* Not of one or other form of disease or class of diseases, but of disease as a whole.

There is, in fact, only one disease.

What appear to us as different disturbances of the normal condition of our body, are only variations, in quantity or in quality, of the one thing. It is the variation of the controlling element which performs the necessary work of keeping the existing cells in proper condition and replacing those which in the course of nature are destroyed. In a word, the work of *perpetual regeneration, which is life.*

METABOLISM.

This continuous changing of the entire human body, — the removal of the discarded cells, burned up by oxidation and expelled from the body in the urine, the perspiration and other excretions, and their replacement by new ones, — is called metabolism, that is, "change of matter."

This change is brought about by means of a vital fluid in the body, which circulates from the moment in which the spermatozoon, or male seed, touches the female egg in the womb of the mother, until the time of our last breath. That fluid is *the blood*, — the carrier of nature's supplies to all parts of the body for the rebuilding of cells; the exact and equitable distributor in quantities of material which determines the quality of the cells.

In its marvelous performance of this function, the blood is the bearer of the sole existing condition of health; namely the necessary elements of cell-building in the right proportions.

This is health, and the lack thereof is disease.

The demand of nature for upbuilding and rebuilding is the strongest instinctive impulse of our being; and this being so, a wrong proportion may cause the upbuilding of things which are different and disturbing to the normal organism.

But, on the other hand, kindly nature exhibits an ever existent inclination to counterbalance any disturbance in the right proportion, and to bring back conditions to uniformity.

We may thus justly speak of *the overwhelming healing tendency of nature*.

Metabolism is, therefore, the one great dominant function of the body which, accordingly, must have our especial care.

It is the blood, consequently, to which alone we can resort if we desire to assist nature in its process and tendency of balancing and healing.

This again indicates that, notwithstanding the apparent great variety of *constitutional diseases, they are all practically one and the same disease. They are all disturbances of proper metabolism, by some irregularity of the quantitative or qualitative condition of the blood.*

This governing truth the great physiologist, Prof. Jacob Moleschott, has formulated in the memorable words: "It is one of the chief questions which humanity must always ask of the physician: how to attain good, healthy and active blood. And, view the question as we may, all who give it serious thought, are forced by experience to acknowledge explicitly, or otherwise, that *our mental and physical capacity, and likewise the power of reproduction, are directly dependent upon our blood, and our blood on our nutrition.*"

VARIETY OF ORGANS.

Why then, you may ask, if such unity exists, why this dissimilarity in the tissues of the respective bodily organs? How is it that a bone in its stonelike hardness is essentially the same as the infinitely tender tissues of the eye? This difference is due to and accounted for by the adaptation of certain portions of the immense accumulation of cells to diverse functions, which has necessitated the variable conformity of the supporting elements. But all of these elements are in the blood, which carries them in the necessary quantities to the different organs to which they belong and where they are utilized to replace used-up matter.

I do not overlook the difficulty of grasping this idea of unity.

The fact, that it is so difficult to realize, has led to the greatest errors in present day medical science.

It seemed at first sight, so obviously necessary to study the different organs as entirely different groups, to work out a careful system of bones, of intestinal organs, of blood-vessels, of nerves, and so on; all of which is of course very valuable, in its place, but only from a descriptive standpoint.

Anatomy shows us what life has produced in the construction of a human form, but it does not indicate the source of life, nor, consequently, the source of health.

It is well to know the different forms of cell accumulations, which are called organs, but if we desire to keep them in good order, we must watch closely what is common to them all; for it is only from this point of view, that we are able to determine the necessary, and possibly, the lacking elements for purposes of healing.

Thus, as one of the greatest achievements of modern science, we come to the one most vital thing, so sorely needed and yet so badly neglected throughout the centuries: *The chemical analysis of the human body and its different organs.*

A new light has now dawned upon the subject most essential to the inauguration of a new and effective system of healing.

The physiological chemist has at length discovered that the human body, and every organ of that body consists of a certain number of chemical elements, which appear in different parts in different aggregations. These aggregations, however, repeat themselves in the various parts or organs.

It was thus finally discovered that there are *twelve different main aggregations of such elements*, which groups of equal elements we call *tissues*.

Through this discovery we have arrived at the great truth that *it is not to the purpose, in healing, to turn attention to the various organs, but rather to the various tissues*.

The influence which can be exercised on these tissues is exercised through the blood which nourishes all of them alike, and which has the wonderful capacity of carrying to each of them their necessary building and rebuilding, or regenerating materials,—*provided, of course, that these are, as they should be, present in the blood.*

THE CONSTITUENT ELEMENTS.

Research in physiological chemistry, has so far determined that there are sixteen definite and discernible elements — and a seventeenth is now in course of determination — which, in their various combinations and aggregations, form the different tissues of which the various organs of the human body are constructed.

The preponderance of one or more of these elements in a certain tissue forms the main or governing feature, or tissue of any organ. Thus the prevalence of potassium phosphate forms the muscle tissue, the prevalence of ammonium phosphate (lecithin) forms the nerve tissue.

For the purpose of general explanation it is sufficient to know that each of the various tissues consist of some of these elements, and that each of the tissues, at whatever part of the body it exists, is affected by the lack of any one of these elements.

The greatest chemist of the age, Justus von Liebig, maintains that if one of the necessary elements in a chemical composition is missing, the rest cannot fulfil their duties, and the consequence of such deficiency is that the cell in question must become diseased and degenerate.

This discovery, known as "the law of the minimum," has thrown an additional reassuring light upon the practice of the new school of medicine.

To bring to the tissue the lacking constituent element or elements by way of the blood is the only means of regenerating that tissue, that is, of healing its diseased cells.

DYSAEMIA THE CAUSE OF ALL CONSTITU-TIONAL DISEASES.

Within the limits of this abstract I do not propose to deal with the disturbances in the system caused by traumatic influences, such as wounds, etc. We are treating only of *constitutional* diseases which, whether of acute or of chronic character, are all caused by the lack of such chemical elements as described.

It has been shown that the blood supplies all the chemical substances to the different tissues, and that, consequently, it is the lack of these elements in the blood, which causes the tissues to degenerate, or, in other words, *the lack of certain chemical elements in the blood is disease.*

It is, therefore, merely a question as to *which of the elements are missing or which do not exist in correct proportion*, that determines the different forms of disease.

When once this fact is established, the method of healing consists mainly in supplying in the regular way, that is, *by certain additions to the regular food*, the missing chemical elements in organic form; and medical science has but *to determine which elements are wanting*, and consequently, must be supplied.

It goes without saying that in this system the old, pernicious drug method of filling the body with various poisons to counteract the effects or symptoms of disease, has no place whatever. Certain poisonous drugs may prove effective to suppress certain symptoms by benumbing the nerves and preventing pain; they may, and do counteract the natural process by which nature exercises her power in various ways in the spontaneous effort to throw off disease, in the form of inflammations, fevers or pains; *but they can never heal, or eradicate disease.*

With the discovery of dysaemia as the governing cause of disease, another idol of regular medicine has been cast down.

Since the discovery of the bacillus or microbe, which in varied form accompanies nearly every variety of disease, it has become a dogma of the at present dominant school of medicine that the various bacilli are the actual causes of the different varieties of disease, and the tendency has been to find some poison that would kill the bacilli in order to heal the disease.

The truth is that the bacillus is not the cause, but the effect of disease; in fact is nothing but another consequence or symptom of a specific form of disease. Bacilli grow spontaneously in the ready soil which the diseased and decomposing tissues provide, through lack of the necessary chemical elements; but to attempt to exterminate them, while the underlying conditions for their reproduction remain unchanged, can, of course, never bring about healing.

And thus the high hopes and claims attached to the sero-therapy inocculation process, the injection into the blood of anti-toxins prepared with the serum of animals, have positively vanished.

Hundreds of thousands of human beings have perished in the course of this delusion; but countless numbers will have cause, yet in our day, to rejoice at the exposure of the stupid and unnatural theory, so long legally enforced, that the introduction into the human system of such poisonous substances could remove or overcome the natural consequences of constitutional disease.

HEREDITY.

The discovery that a diseased condition of the blood leads to certain bodily disturbances which we call disease, was soon followed by the realization of the fact that one of the main conditions which bring about such disturbances is predisposition, which in many cases is hereditary.

"Hereditary disease" simply means that the improper chemical composition of the blood of one or both parents has become duplicated in the offspring, and that it has similar consequences in causing the degeneration of certain tissues, and consequently of the organs composed thereof, as may have been the case in the parents.

It is at least reassuring to know, however, *that to the modern hygienic-dietetic system of healing, heredity, though perhaps more tenacious, is by no means an invincible enemy.*

With a predisposition to disease the child acquires also the hereditary tendency to self-protection, and thus rational hygienic-dietetic treatment may be able to eliminate, in a comparatively short time, the chain of diseases which in former years, generations have carried hopelessly to the grave.

HEALING.

It has been already stated that healing, under the modern hygienic-dietetic system, means supplying to the blood such chemical elements as will replace what are missing in defective tissues of the body.

I will now outline the methods of carrying it into effect.

In a general way there are three means of doing this:

No. 1. *Diet*: The first and most natural way is by proper diet.

As the normal chemical elements are introduced into the body as constituents of the regular daily food, the task which, in the first place, confronts the hygienic-dietetic physician is that of regulating the quantity, quality and description of food.

Too little importance has heretofore been given to this question and, beyond prohibiting certain dishes and obviously detrimental viands, little attention was paid by the average physician to the matter of the every-day nourishment of the patient.

The hygienic-dietetic physician on the other hand, employs the utmost care in giving to the patient everything that will help to regenerate his blood, laying particular stress on such foods as contain the largest proportion of the chemical elements that are missing in the affected tissues.

No. 2. *Nutritive compositions*: The process of destruction, however, which has to be met, in more or less advanced stages, in nearly every case requires supply, in quantity of the pure material to compensate the deficiency of the missing elements, beyond that which could be derived in the ordinary way of digestion from every-day food.

To meet this difficulty, certain condensed preparations have been devised.

These nutritive compositions contain only such chemical elements in like chemical proportions as exist in the human body. They are of the purest material and contain no injurious elements whatsoever, while they foster that general regeneration of the blood which will finally bring about a complete cure.

No. 3. *Physical treatments*: It is the object of these treatments to assist the proper circulation of the blood; to automatically open the pores of the skin for the external treatment of certain diseases; to withdraw elements of disease from the body, and to introduce certain material influences, through the pores.

Massage, gymnastics, ablutions, various kinds of baths and "packs," constitute the chief features of the healing methods in this department.

Following this general explanation of the system, I may now go a little deeper into the question of the constituent elements, the tissues formed therefrom, the degeneration of these tissues, and the species of degeneration which constitutes the various forms of disease commonly known to us.

After this I will give a concise and simple general idea as to how my methods should be applied.

THE UNITY OF NATURE.

To fully understand the method of healing which I apply, it is necessary to understand one of the great natural laws, the discovery of which by the great chemists, Justus von Liebig and Julius Hensel, has shown us the path along which to proceed.

This law demonstrates that, in the last analysis, *nature is a unit, a composition of a number of elements, each one possessing distinct qualities, the combination of which produces the various manifestations of life*.

These are classified, for convenience, according to their main qualities, as minerals, plants or animals.

All of them are closely interrelated and one transmits the basic elements to the other. It is the plant which draws the mineral elements from the soil, and after certain processes of composition conveys them as food to the animal, including the human being, while such animal substances as are used for human food, contribute the balance of the elements for the upbuilding of the human body.

It is a matter of comparatively new discovery that minerals are thus just as important as a component part of the body and of its food as are other basic chemical elements.

The discovery as to the mineral constituents of the body, their nature, proportion and in which composition and in which quantity as necessary ingredients of the different body tissues, in order that they may become a part of the organism, has made it possible to administer them to the diseased body in the purest condensed and most effective way in *nutritive compositions*, while their proportionate existence in food is also a criterion of diet, not only for the sick, but also as a preventative of disease.

THE CHEMICAL PROCESS OF DISEASE.

In this, my scrutiny of nature's deep designs, I did not rest content when only the composition of all the tissues of the body had been laid bare; but I delved deeper and discovered that certain electric currents and reactions of these elements were the causes of accelerating or retarding the natural processes of metamorphosis and metabolism,—provoking disturbances of the normal, which express themselves as disease.

Excessive growth, and lack of growth, are thus explained, together with other phenomena which in this short chapter it is impossible to give in scientific detail. It is my object now merely to show that in their apparent simplicity the manifestations of life require special technical knowledge such as cannot be expected of the layman in any adequate degree.

Notwithstanding this free and open statement of cause and cure available to the patient and to the world at large, the hygienic-dietetic physician himself can by no means be dispensed with in case of the appearance of disease, for only by his knowledge, experience, and skilled advice can the aforesaid natural system of healing be applied with effect in each individual case. And here it must always be borne in mind that, of the countless individual organisms that this world contains, no two, even, are exactly alike; and that consequently only the skilled and accustomed practitioner **will be able to regulate such hidden, internal processes as cause the visible disturbance, and thus bring about healing and regeneration, which simply means a return to the normal.**

His methods will prevent the use of the surgeon's knife, which only removes the symptom, leaving the cause untouched and inflicting useless and irreparable harm. The specialist, with his poisonous specific remedies for forms of disease, which after all are only degrees of chemical exhaustion, will also disappear, together with all similar treatment which enervates the body making it an easy prey to new attacks of the same chemical anomalies which must and will most certainly return so long as they are not rectified according to the principles of biology.

THE TWELVE TISSUES.

Bearing the above principle of unity in mind, we may now proceed one step further, and study the most important details upon which the method of healing, as applied by the hygienic-dietetic physician, is based.

As previously mentioned, the cells of the human body are organized into twelve distinct tissues, some of which are the component parts of the various organs as discernible by form and function.

These twelve tissues are the following:

1. The plasmo tissue (blood plasma).
2. The lymphoid tissue.
3. The nerve tissue.
4. The bone tissue.
5. The muscular tissue.
6. The mucous membrane tissue.
7. The tooth and eye tissue.
8. The hair tissue.
9. The skin tissue.
10. The gelatigenous tissue.
11. The cartilage tissue.
12. The body tissue in general.

1. *The plasmo tissue*: This tissue is a liquid, the blood plasma, which is one of the important component parts of the life-giving substance, blood. It is the blood serum—blood-water and fibrogen—which harbours the white and the red corpuscles. The red corpuscles are the carriers of oxygen to the various tissues, which the body draws from the atmosphere, and of the other nutriments. They exchange it for the carbonic acid which is forming in the body, and while the blood in flowing through the system of arteries, brings the oxygen, it carries away, through the veins, the poisonous carbonic acid which is exhaled into the atmosphere.

The red corpuscles, after having performed their duties, enter the liver and are used to build the gall.

The proper quality of the plasma alone regulates the speed of blood circulation and ensures its entrance into the finest capillaries — the ultimate branches of the blood-vessels — hence, its capacity to carry supplies of nutriment to the tissues. The disturbance of this proper quality is among the main factors of constitutional disease.

2. *The lymphoid tissue*: The lymph is another of the life-giving liquids of the body, which through a vascular system of its own, draws certain nutritive substances from the food and carries them to certain organs which it feeds, especially the nerves.

After this slow task is completed, the rest of the lymph enters the blood and is carried by it to other parts of the body where only smaller quantities of lymph are needed for nourishing purposes.

The proper quality and chemical composition of the lymph, which is different from that of the blood, is of no less importance than that of the plasma for the preservation and regeneration of the organism.

What the plasma is to the blood, the lymph is to the nerves.

3. *The nerve tissue*: A particular aggregation of cells forms the nerves, which, emanating from their center in the brain and spine, run as another separate system all through the body.

This system, however, is not one of vessels; but the nerves may best be compared to the wires of a telephone system, establishing connection between the remotest parts of the body and its central point, from which the directions for both voluntary and involuntary movement are given and transmitted through the nerves.

They are of a peculiar chemical composition in which the nerve fat (lecithin) plays a very important part, since its frequent presence in insufficient quantity is among the most common causes of a great number of nervous and other diseases.

4. *The bone tissue*: The bones consist of a special and very distinct tissue in which lime predominates. This gives them the strength and solidity which enables them to act as support to all the other organs.

The bones too are fed by the blood, and it is through the blood that the necessary constituent parts for the regeneration of their tissue is conveyed to them.

While naturally their power of resistance is greater than that of any other organ, they are nevertheless subject to a number of structural disturbances, other than traumatic, the causes of which are sometimes hereditary, sometimes acquired through deficient properties of the nourishing blood.

Certain tissues which form the connection between the bones and the rest of the organs, and the gradual transition into other tissues, are subjects separate and distinct and will be treated separately.

5. *The muscular tissue*: As to quantity, the muscular tissue represents the maximum of any in the human body.

The muscles do not only consist solely of this one tissue, but of several others, as do most of the other organs; but here, as in all other cases, the principal component element is called after the organ in which it is chiefly found.

The structure of the muscular tissue varies according to its function, so that we distinguish between the striated and the unstriated or smooth muscles. This, however, has no influence on their chemical composition, a distinctive element of which is muscular fibrin, which has the particular property of contractibility.

6. *The mucous membrane tissue*: The mucous membrane forms the covering of many of the organs, and its chemical and structural composition is identical in all parts of the body.

It is characterized by a viscid watery secretion from the mucous glands, which are always found in the mucous membrane.

Its extremely delicate nature renders it subject to all sorts of irregularities in chemical composition.

This is the cause of numerous diseases, most of which are due either to overproduction or underproduction of the secretion which regulates numerous functions of the body.

7. *The tooth and eye tissue*: While very different in external appearance, functions and physical qualities, the teeth and the eyes have nevertheless, the most important part of their chemical composition in common; namely, *the fluoric acid*, which distinguishes them from all other tissues.

In the process of natural healing the replacing of any element lacking through destructive causes in either tissue will practically be the same.

8. *The hair tissue*: Certain chemical component elements are only found in the tissue which is called the hair, and which receives its nourishment like all other tissues, through the blood.

While the hair may seem to be in apparently slight connection with the rest of the body, it is in reality, none the less an organic portion of the same, and dependent, like the rest upon the same central system of supply.

9. *The skin tissue*: With reference to this tissue, much the same remarks apply as already mentioned in regard to the mucous membrane. It, however, has certain chemical elements, which are characteristic to its various layers.

Since the skin forms the most important intermediary between the external elements and the chemical and structural elements of the interior of the human body, it is of the greatest importance that its chemical composition should always be correct, and that it should not be subject to decomposition such as improper nourishment engenders.

It should be borne in mind that the skin, like all other organs of the body, grows from the inside outward, so that any ailment concerning the skin, which is not of a traumatic nature, must be based upon wrong or insufficient nourishment, and cannot be cured in any other way than by internal regenerative means.

10. *The gelatigenous tissue*: This tissue, chemically and otherwise peculiar as it is, forms the chief component part of many of the human organs, and it may be truly said that the lack of attention which its peculiarities have received in the past is responsible for more disease and its fatal issue than almost anything else.

The gelatigenous tissue contains a number of special component elements, which require special nourishment through proper diet; and in view of the fact that the gelatigenous tissue pervades so many of the various organs, its effect upon the functional abilities of a great number of them is obvious.

The elasticity of most organs which work by contraction and expansion, depends entirely upon the gelatigenous, rubber-like tissue of which they are so largely composed.

11. *The cartilage tissue*: Practically the same applies to the cartilage tissue; but it is only recently that it has been found to what extent this is the case.

Although entirely different in nature and chemical composition, the cartilage tissue serves to maintain certain outlines of form and feature in the human body, which are not based on the still stronger forms of supporting material, such as the bone tissue and the gelatigenous tissue.

12. *The body tissue in general*: This comprises the red blood corpuscles and all tissues which are in any way different from the distinct tissues just described, but which nevertheless cannot be classified as separately and distinctly independent.

It may be justly presumed that all elements of the other tissues are to be found in these final tissues which share the unity of the organism.

By devising a specially nourishing dietary system for the body tissue in general, all component elements profit, in like degree, and such disturbances as attack practically all the tissues and organs of the body severally and conjointly; will be effectively prevented or cured in the regular course of nature, in strict accordance with biological principles.

DEGENERATION OF TISSUES.

Speaking biologically, if through some disturbance in the normal chemical composition of the tissues, degeneration sets in, we speak of it as disease.

Such degeneration may attack one tissue or several at the same time.

To reduce the elements to their proper proportions, to force them thereby to reassume their normal functions, means to restore health, or, to heal.

As previously explained, it has been the great achievement of hygienic-dietetic science, based on the natural laws of biology, to discover that so many diseases which for centuries were considered as entirely different from each other in cause and treatment, were essentially the same. It was found that they were nothing but the natural consequence of impure or imperfect blood, the result of malnutrition of the vital fluid, the malign effect of which increases in degree and manifestation the longer the impurity passes, by process of heredity, from one generation to another.

Instead of following the natural tendency to return to the normal, the blood becomes the fertile soil in which all manner of irregularities may germinate in abundance, and combine in strong attacks on the normal healthy organs, which will fast relax their natural power of resistance.

The system of natural healing, while adhering closely to the principle of the unity of the body as well as of the unity of disease, has by no means ignored that such differences are due to the differences in the twelve tissues and *according to the said differences, the constitutional diseases are grouped under the accustomed titles, as follows*:

1. Degeneration of the plasmo tissue: Anaemia, Chlorosis, Pernicious Anaemia, etc. (A.) Scrofulosis. (B.) Tuberculosis. (C.) Syphilis. (D.) Cancer.

2. Degeneration of lymphoid tissue: (See I. — A. B. C. D.)

3. Degeneration of the nerve tissue: Neuralgia, Neuritis, Neurasthenia, Asthma, Epilepsy, St. Vitus's Dance, etc., etc.

4. Degeneration of the bone tissue: Rickets, Osteomalacia and similar diseases.

5. Degeneration of the muscular tissue: Muscular Rheumatism, Sciatica or Nerve Rheumatism, Atrophia, Amyloid heart, kidney and liver.

6. Degeneration of the mucous membrane tissue. (A.) Catarrh in all its forms: Bronchitis, Pleurisy, Pneumonia, Inflammation of nose, throat, bowels, stomach, bladder, etc. (B.) Hemorrhoids, Polyps, Adenoids.

7. Degeneration of the tooth and eye tissue: All tooth and eye diseases.

8. Degeneration of the hair tissue: All hair diseases.

9. Degeneration of the skin tissue: All skin diseases.

10. Degeneration of the gelatigenous tissue. (A.) Stomach and Intestinal diseases—acute forms. (B.) Stomach and Intestinal diseases—chronic form.

11. Degeneration of the cartilage tissue: Ankylosis, Gout, Arthritis deformans.

12. Degeneration of the body tissue in general.
(A.) Locomotor ataxia. (B.) Basedow's disease. (Graves disease.) (C.) Diabetes mellitus. (D.) Obesity. (E.) Bright's disease. (F.) Arterio-sclerosis.

THE A.B.C. OF MY SYSTEM OF HEALING.

Setting aside for the time being the special groups of more complicated diseases, such as are characterized by the degeneration of several of the tissues at the same time, I will now give a short and comprehensive description of the several distinct groups of disease. In each case, as already shown, there must be a joint co-operation of these three factors:

(A.) *Diet*, or the natural means of providing both healthy and degenerating tissues alike with such substances as will support and strengthen the healthy tissues, enabling them to resist the danger of disease and consequent decomposition, and will also arrest degeneration and prepare the way for the regeneration of the tissue which is already affected.

(B.) *Nutritive compositions*. Such as will in each case introduce into the system in a pure and proportionate combination, the necessary quantities of the sixteen nutritive elements, the lack of which is the characteristic factor of all disease and which diet unaided could not adequately produce with the needful speed and proportion, unless supplemented in this simple and effective manner.

(C.) *Physical treatment*, for the purpose of assisting the proper distribution and assimilation of these nutritive factors — (A. and B.) — and promoting the proper circulation of the blood.

DIET.

This is a subject of vast and vital importance. It comprises the science of alimentation, which forms one of the indispensable functions of life; it is thus, of necessity, a serious preoccupation under all conditions.

I have treated this important subject in my greater work with the minute detail, which it deserves; thus, in following the advice given, therein, in chapter XVIII, the reader will be able to ascertain the foods that are best suited to various conditions, and how to prepare them in the most sensible way.

At present, I can treat it only in a short and general way, giving the principal groups of diet prescribed, with more or less variation, in each case of disease as a part of the general treatment.

A few words may show *why* diet plays so important a part in this system of healing.

In the body there is a laboratory which produces spontaneously everything necessary to maintain life.

This laboratory has various branches which are busy day and night without interruption.

Here the life blood is created.

Prominent amongst these branches are:

The stomach with its prolonged intestines;
The liver;
The kidneys;
The lungs, and
The skin.

Each one of these branches has a distinct part, or function to perform.

The stomach serves as the sorting house. Here the food is mixed with the gastric juice which aids digestion and dissolves those ingredients necessary to produce blood, flesh, fat, bones, etc.

Each of the other branches receives that portion of the ingredients needed to perform its share of the work.

A structure cannot be constructed without a frame upon which every part depends. In order to stand erect, the body must possess such a framework. The skeleton is the same to the body as the frame is to the building. This frame, then, or skeleton, together with the flesh, blood, etc. are all formed from the material furnished by the food.

A residue of the digested food is removed from the body as useless; everything else is utilized.

The portion of the food used, therefore, must contain all those ingredients which go to make up and maintain the body in perfect working order.

Experience has suggested certain groups of suitable diet which for the sake of convenience I shall enumerate under the title of *Forms No. I to No. VI.*

These food forms contain everything of which patients may safely partake, and from these selection, in each case, must be made.

They are as follows:

Form I. Complete elimination of the stomach in the nourishing process.

To allay thirst, moisten the mouth with pure or carbonized water, melting small pieces of ice on the tongue. Small sips of water either lukewarm or cold, according to the condition of the stomach. Otherwise, only introduce water by clyster—i.e.—injection, and if the stomach cannot be disturbed for more than one or two days, introduce nourishing substances by way of the rectum.

Form II. Purely liquid nourishment, "soup diet."

Consommé of pigeon, chicken, veal, mutton, beef, beef tea, meat jelly (which becomes liquid under the influence of the heat of the body,) strained soups or such as are prepared of the finest flour with water or bouillon, of barley, oats, rice (thick soup), green corn, rye flour, malted milk. All of these soups, with or without any additions, such as raw eggs, either whole or the yolk only, if well mixed and not coagulated, are easily digested.

Form III. Nourishment which is not purely liquid, but partly glutinous.

Milk and milk preparations (belonging to this group on account of their coagulation in the stomach):

(a) Cow's milk, diluted and without cream, dilution with 1-2 to 2-3 barley water, rice water, lime water, vichy water, weak tea, or pure water.

(b) Milk without cream, not diluted.

(c) Unskimmed milk.

(d) Cream, either diluted or undiluted.

(e) All of these milk combinations with an addition of yolk of egg, well-mixed, whole egg, cocoa, also a combination of egg and cocoa.

Milk mush made of flour for children, arrowroot, mondanin, cereal flour of every kind, especially oats, groat soups with tapioca or sago and potato soup.

Egg,-raw, stirred, or sucked from the shell; or slightly warmed in a cup; any of these, either with or without the addition of a little sugar or salt.

Biscuit and crackers, softened or well masticated and salivated, taken with milk, mush, etc.

Form IV. Diet of the lightest kind, containing meat, but still mainly glutinous.

Noodle soup, rice soup.

Mashed boiled brains or sweetbread, or puree of white or red roasted meat, in soup.

Brains and sweetbread boiled.

Raw scraped meat (beef, ham, etc.)

Lean veal sausages, boiled.

Mashed potatoes prepared with milk.

Rice with bouillon or with milk.

Toasted rolls and toast.

Form V. Light diet, containing meat in more solid form:

Pigeon, Chicken boiled.

Small fish with little fat, such as brook or lake trout, boiled.

Scraped beefsteak, raw ham, boiled tongue.

As delicacies: Small quantities of caviar, frogs' legs, oysters, sardelles softened in milk.

Salted potatoes crushed, spinach, young peas mashed, cauliflower, asparagus-tips, mashed chestnuts, mashed turnips, fruit sauces.

Groat or sago puddings.

Rolls, white bread.

Form VI. Somewhat heavier meat diet. (Gradually returning to ordinary food).

Pigeon, chicken, young deer, hare, everything roasted.

Beef tenderloin, tender roast beef, roast veal.

Boiled pike or carp.

Young turnips.

All dishes to be prepared with very little fat, butter to be used exclusively. All strong spices to be avoided.

NOTE:—For special dietary in all diseases, see under each separate tissue degeneration in the succeeding Chapter on Therapy.

FOOTNOTES:

[A] In the following chapter, several important paragraphs given in the foregoing had to be repeated as the readers who were not interested in the "Club" proposition, would miss these points.

NUTRITIVE COMPOSITIONS

In order to convey a better understanding of these nutritive compositions, I deem it necessary to outline and explain more emphatically and in greater detail their wonderful scope and possibilities, in perhaps a more impressive manner, by giving the reader the benefit of an article entitled:

> "The functions of minerals in our food
> How they may be greatly increased"

Of these I have sent some 560 copies to all our Senators and Congressmen, as well as to our chief Government Physicians, for their information and disposition, with the intention of placing my knowledge and equipment freely at the disposal of the United States Government. I have made this purely disinterested proposal at this critical and trying juncture, in the interest, first, of our war-worn soldiers; next, of our women, enervated by unaccustomed labour and restricted means; and lastly, of the children, born, and yet to be born of them—the future Citizens of the Republic—all, in short, who, under stress of injury, strain and hardship abroad, or the sometimes equally strenuous privations of war conditions at home, may, in their respective degrees, be suffering from nervous breakdown or depleted vitality and the various disorders which my proffered remedial measures are so admirably fitted to successfully overcome, bearing, as they must untold relief, comfort and renewed health to thousands.

I have not spared expense in putting this matter fairly and fully before the Authorities—and indeed the initial cost of so doing has already absorbed some $300 or more. That is merely a detail. But the main point is this: That I have offered this valuable knowledge—

(practically the work of a lifetime) — to the Nation, together with the prescriptions of my compositions, free of cost, as an earnest of my sympathy and goodwill; and had the Government, seen fit to accept my proposal, the immediate effect would have been that these compounds, which at present, through reduced manufacture and the consequent great scarcity of chemicals (necessarily of the finest description and purity) are very costly, would have been brought by extensive and organized production within the reach of every citizen, removing at once that paramount difficulty of my system, so far as the general public is concerned; namely, the expense.

I append hereto a copy of the article referred to, together with copy of an accompanying letter.

My dear Senator:

The disarrangement of the habits of life of our civilian population, and the physical needs of our boys who will return from Europe wounded and crippled, prompts me to offer my services to the Government for the development of specially enriched foodstuffs to maintain the health of our people under the strain of the war, but particularly to aid in the speedy recovery of our boys who return shattered from the trenches. I have spent more than thirty years in the study of physiological chemistry and biology, and this study has been devoted to the application of scientific principles in the treatment of various diseases.

Hitherto our food experts and medical men have been satisfied with a ration properly balanced as regards protein, carbohydrates and fat, but the mineral salts in our food have been given little if any serious consideration. Indeed, they have usually been dismissed as "ash." As a matter of fact, however, as the statement I am sending you under separate cover will show clearly, even to a layman, mineral salts perform an important function in keeping the body strong and healthy.

I am prepared to demonstrate that the quantity of essential minerals in vegetables, small fruit and eggs can be multiplied several times by scientific fertilization and nutrition. If I can do this (and I am prepared to prove that I can) the Government should be willing to arrange for the production of such foods in connection with every military hospital and convalescent camp, both here at home and behind the lines in Europe. Moreover, given a central experimental station with proper equipment, it would be an easy matter to train men to teach this knowledge to soldiers at every reconstruction camp.

The statement is made by Dr. Mae H. Cardwell, of Portland, Oregon, one of the investigators for the Federal Children's Bureau that millions of children are suffering from lack of sufficient food and from improper feeding, and she adds that not only the parents but the doctors, in many cases, need education with respect to what constitutes proper feeding for children. I think that when you have read and digested my statement of the function of the mineral salts in the human economy, you will agree with me that the need for just what I am asking the government to give me an opportunity of doing is very great indeed.

I trust that I may count upon your co-operation, not only in getting this matter before the proper officials, but also in seeing that an opportunity for a fair demonstration is accorded me.

The dissemination of this knowledge and the production of such foods would make America the ALMA MATER of the world in scientific nutrition, thanks to the application of physiological chemistry. As things are now done in agriculture and in aviculture, however, very little can be expected along this line.

I will give you two concrete illustrations of what can be done in the way of augmenting the mineral content of food, and then I will point out the significance of that fact. We will consider eggs: ordinarily 100 grams of egg yolk contains from 10 to 20 milligrams of iron, but eggs laid by hens fed by my method yield from 30 to 80 milligrams of iron per 100 grams of dried yolk. This is an increase, as you see, of between 300 and 400 per cent. Such eggs might be justly classed as haemoglobin eggs, and they would be a godsend to our boys suffering from anaemia due to wounds or operations. At the same time, my method of handling chickens greatly enriches the lecithin, or nerve substance, in the eggs, and they are, therefore, of special value in dealing with cases of shell shock and nerve exhaustion.

What is true in the case of iron and lecithin content of eggs produced by my method, is equally true with respect to their content of all the other essential mineral elements; they are all multiplied several times.

This is made possible of accomplishment by the application of the principles of physiological chemistry to the breeding and feeding of the poultry.

Needless to say, I am prepared to submit to the test of scientific examination of my claims. No, not merely a theoretical examination of myself, but, rather, to submit the claim I make for eggs produced under my direction to the test of chemical analysis. It is a very easy matter to determine thereby whether my claims are well founded.

I cannot state my desire to serve the government in this way too strongly; as I have spent more than thirty years of my life in the study of biology and physiological chemistry, I feel that it is my duty to offer to the Government the benefits of my knowledge and experience. All that I can ask in this connection is to be given an opportunity to prove that my claims are sound and practical.

I believe that you will realize the full value of such a course of action as outlined, if it can be proven practicable. The opportunity of offering proof under direction of the proper branch of government is, I repeat, all that I ask at the moment, as the results will tell their own story far more eloquently than mere words.

Thanking you for giving this matter your attention, and trusting that my hope of serving in the ranks of those seeking to rebuild our boys will not prove vain, I am, Sir,

Yours truly,

L. DECHMANN.

THE FUNCTION OF MINERALS IN OUR FOOD:

HOW THEY MAY BE GREATLY INCREASED.
By LOUIS DECHMANN.
1918.

When physiological chemistry has isolated and classified the component elements of the various organs, tissues and fluids of the body, it must analyze and classify the vegetables, fruits and meats on which man feeds in order that we may not only know how to arrange a perfectly balanced ration for the healthy, but shall be able to add lacking elements to the diet of the diseased. This classification of foods naturally leads, if there be a deficiency of any essential element, to the analysis of the soil on which this food was raised.

In the course of my studies in physiological chemistry and biology, which have extended over a period of more than thirty years, I have been led to grapple with problems in agriculture, in horticulture, and in aviculture, for the purpose of finding solutions to problems in human nutrition. Very early in my studies I learned the value of the mineral elements in our foodstuffs. I was led to attempt to augment the quantity of mineral salts in various foods, and my efforts were crowned with success. But this is not the point, however, to enter into a detailed discussion of that aspect of the subject.

It may be wise for the sake of clearness to divide this statement into two parts, as follows:

1. A brief summary of the function of minerals in the human economy.

2. A short argument showing how we can and why it is imperative that we should augment the mineral content of our vegetables, small fruits and eggs.

In the case of eggs, for example, I am able to increase their iron content 300 or 400 per cent. More than that, I can multiply every item in their mineral content several times, thus producing specific eggs for those suffering for lack of any mineral. In other words I am able to produce special eggs for a given tissue degeneration as, for instance, haemoglobin eggs for degenerate blood; lecithin eggs for the nerves; calcareous eggs for the bones, and kaliated eggs for the muscle.

So much by way of preface.

I.

The following explanations are made for the purpose of showing you that I have made extensive studies along these lines, and are not, naturally, intended to be taken as a lesson to you personally.

There are sixteen chemical elements absolutely essential to healthy human life, which are classified by physiological chemistry as the elements of organic life. In the composition of vital tissues we constantly find these basal elements: Carbon, oxygen, hydrogen, nitrogen, sulphur, phosphorus, chlorine, potassium, sodium, magnesium, calcium, iron, manganese, fluorine, silicon, and iodine. The function of these elements will be discussed in a moment.

I would here lay stress upon the fact that the absence of the tiniest ingredient necessary to the growth and functioning of an organ will, according to the Law of the Minimum as laid down by Justus von Liebig, result in disease, improper functioning and degeneration of that organ or tissue.

Although the chemical salts constitute but a small part in the composition of our bodies, and are a very small item in our daily diet, their importance cannot be too strongly emphasized. They are the main sources for the development of electro-magnetic energy in the blood and nerves, and perform other services. I am of the opinion that "vitamines" are neither more or less than these chemicals in proper proportion and relation, but whether you agree or disagree with this conclusion, you will instantly agree that the elements named above are indispensible to perfect metabolism.

It goes without saying, of course, that no action in the world occurs of itself, that is without impulse, hence the body must be given impulse to growth. A series of chemical and physical facts indicate that phosphorus plays this vital part. The property of phosphoric acid of uniting with carburetted hydrogen to form carbonic acid and phosphureted hydrogen certainly is of fundamental importance, as phosphureted hydrogen readily ignites on coming into contact with oxygen. Since cerebrin consists of a combination of phosphoric acid with gelatine which contains ammonium and with oleine, it is easy to infer that the light of the soul may be due to the phosphoric acid in the nerves, and still further the potassium phosphate forming the mineral basis of the muscles. Thus we come to the conclusion that the phosphates, combinations of phosphoric acid with basic substances, possess in general the property of imparting the true impulse to growth, that is to accumulation of organic matter.

Like every other structure, however, the body requires supports and props and, above all, a firm foundation on which to rest. Iron and lime, whose union is secured by their opposition to one another, bring into conjunction materials of contrary disposition for the creating of organic forms of the nature of plant and animal bodies.

The sulphuric compounds are related and yet opposed to the growth determining phosphoric compounds. All organic building material (protein) contains phosphorus and sulphur, in varying proportions, and all indications are that sulphur plays the part of a regulator in organic growth. Just as an engine requires a governor to regulate its pace, so the human body requires a controlling factor to ensure definite stability. It is interesting to observe that normal blood contains about twice as many sulphates as phosphates. When there is great scarcity of sodium sulphate in the blood, abnormal growths develop from the phosphatic nerve tissues, and they continue to develop so long as the blood and lymph are deficient in sulphur, particularly the sulphates. This is, I believe, the genesis of polyps, tumors and cancers.

In the same manner that sulphuric acid controls and regulates the phosphoric acid of ammonium phosphate, so lime and magnesia act on the ammonia of this same ammonium phosphate.

Phosphatic ammonium carbonate lodges in the gelatinous cartilage and stretches it, when there is a deficiency of lime and magnesia in the food, resulting in rickets. Such a growth of cartilaginous tissues is controlled by lime and magnesia, as they change the pliant cartilage into bony barriers in which small particles of magnesia combine to produce phosphate of ammonium and magnesium which checks the further deposit of cartilage.

Lime and magnesia are indubitably quite as effective agents in the control of ammonia as sulphur is in the control of phosphorus. If we consider the minerals as the foundation and mortar which give stability to the vital machine, leaving out chlorine and fluorine, we find that iron, manganese, potash, soda, and silicic acid play this role. Sulphur, because it possesses the property of becoming gaseous, is able to take part directly in the formation of albumen, that variable basis of body material, whereas all of the other mineral substances except silicic acid can only be assimiliated in so-called binary compounds in the form of salts.

I will give a brief review of them, beginning with iron, as thus the significance of augmentation of the mineral content of vegetables and small fruits and eggs will be made much clearer.

Normal blood albumen is essentially a compound of calcium and sodium into which iron and sulphur both enter. A deficiency of calcium commonly makes itself known by dental defects, just as lack of sulphur reveals itself by the falling out and poor growth of hair. Insufficiency of iron in the blood is evidenced, apart from lack of spirit, by paleness of face and blue lips; insufficient sodium by glandular tumors and abnormal cartilaginous growths.

The entire amount of iron in the blood of an adult person is, on the average under normal conditions, four grams, as much as a nickel weighs. We may well judge that this amount is not sufficient to set the motive power of our bodies in action, if we overlook that complex factor the circulation of blood. The left side of the heart has the capacity of containing about six ounces of blood, and every heart beat drives this amount through the aorta. With seventy beats to the minute, twenty-five pounds of blood is pumped from the heart every minute. What is the result? That the four grams of iron keep up such an incessant movement that they pass from the heart into the aorta sixty times an hour or 1440 times in 24 hours. It may be asserted, therefore, that in 24 hours 13 pounds of iron (that is 1440x4 grams) pass from the heart into the aorta. Can it be doubted, in view of this, that the iron serves to produce an electro-dynamic force?

In respect to the generation of electricity, it matters not whether there be an entirely new supply of iron passing a given point, or whether the same iron pass that point anew each minute. Two factors work together in the circulation of the blood, namely, the active attraction of nerve tissue and the passive susceptibility of the blood contents to that attraction. Faraday has conclusively shown that blood is magnetic in character because of the iron it contains. If four grams of iron is the normal quantity in the blood, it is clear that the reduction of this amount, say by two grams, will lessen its susceptibility and slacken its circulation. The electrical nerve ends will then strain in vain for the electricity which the blood current should yield, and the result will be neuralgia.

It is the magnetic iron in haemoglobin which makes every sort of nervous function possible, in the cerebral (brain) and in the sympathetic (intestinal) tracts, and since it is thus made clear that intellectual activity on the one hand and breathing and digestion and excretion on the other are dependent on the iron content of the blood, we must also recognize that, as iron attends every nerve action, the secretion of urine too takes place under the influence of haemoglobin. Insofar as haemoglobin hastens the departure of the excrementitious matter in urine out of the system, there is a daily loss of iron in the urine. This loss in the form of urohaematin may total four centigrams, or a hundredth part of our supply.

This loss of iron if not replaced by eating suitable food will soon make itself felt. In the course of a day the reduction by four centigrams will diminish the energy of nervous activity about 1440 times the apparent loss, so that even a four weeks-tropical fever, during which no meat is eaten, may completely exhaust the strength of an individual. Moreover, iron conditions bodily warmth as it combines with oxygen in a higher and a lower degree. In the lungs it is highly oxidized by the respired oxygen, but in contact with the nerve ends it gives itself only to a part of the oxygen present, and burns a certain portion of the lecithin to water, carbonic acid and phosphates, thus creating body warmth to a considerable extent.

In response to the chemical consumption of lecithin a new oil flows down the axis cylinders of the nerve fibrils, which are arranged like lamp wicks. The duration of the flow of this oil is, on the average, about eighteen hours. When the cerebro-spinal nerves refuse longer to perform their function, fatigue and sleep ensue, and the current of blood leaves the brain and seeks the intestines. While the cerebro-spinal system rests, the sympathetic system takes up its task of directing the renewal of tissue and supplying the nerve sheaths through the lymph vessels, which draw their material from the digestive canal, with a new supply of phosphatic oil. Thus the brain and spinal nervous system are prepared for another day's work. For the fulfillment of these processes, the magnetic blood current forms the intermediary.

The presence of formic and acetic acid supplies the blood with fresh electricity to stimulate the nerves. "Under normal conditions," says Julius Hensel, "this function is assigned to the spleen. This organ takes the part of a rejuvenating influence in the body in the manner of a relay station, and does so by virtue of an invisible but significant device. In every other region of the body the hairlike terminals of the arteries which branch out from the heart merge directly in the tiny tubes (capillaries) of the veins, which lead back to the heart again: in the spleen this is not the case. Here rather the arteries end suddenly when they have diminished to a diameter of one one-hundred-and-fortieth of an inch and end in a bulb (the Malpighian bodies). Under such circumstances the sudden stoppage, particularly the impact of the magnetic blood stream against the membrane of a Malpighian body, exemplifies the physical law of the induction of electricity, in accordance with which the blood that enters the spleen is changed into plasma and exudes through the membrane of the Malpighian bodies. The event indicates some fluidity of the red blood cells, which is a change effected in the body by the impact of electric sparks, and one which electrical therapy also brings about locally to prevent increase in the solid constituents of the blood."

The numerous Malpighian bodies in the spleen act as so many electrical conductors, and the product of their electrical activity is found in the formic and acetic acid of the fluid plasma which filters through the Malpighian corpuscles and supplies the acid tissue of the spleen (pulpa splenica). These acids are the electrolytic division products of lecithin. In the splenic pulp arise the capillaries of the splenic veins whose acid blood is carried directly to the liver, where certain cells formed like galvanic elements possess the property, through the electrical action of formic and acetic acid, of extracting from blood albumen the opposite of acids, namely, alkaline bile The normal functioning of the liver, therefore, is dependent upon that of the spleen, and since the bile produced by the liver goes to aid the digestive activity of the duodenum, disturbance of digestion must result when the quality of the bile is inferior.

One of the substances contained in bile, lecithin, is of wide importance. When it was referred to a moment ago, I spoke only of its individual chemical nature as a fat in combination with ammonium phosphate, as by so doing I avoided error in connection with its apparently complicated formula, which includes glycerophosphoric acid, trimethylamin, palmitic and stearic acids. As it is a fatty substance, the only question that arises, is, what does it contain besides fat? This may be answered by a process of substraction:

2 (C_{21} H_{42} O_4) C_{42} H_{84} O_8 which represents tallow or stearate of glycerine. Lecithin, C_{42} H_{84} O_9 NP, differs from this only by a larger amount of NP. The significance of this difference becomes clear when two atoms of water are added. Then ammonium phosphate, PO_3 H_4, N is formed. The two atoms of water needed for the condensation of the ammonium phosphate from the stearate are obtained by separating them away from two of glycerine.

The bile contains lecithin in a partially oxidized form. The chemical "remainders" are biliverdin and cholesterin. The latter when normal has, as you know, the power to neutralize snake venoms and other poisons, and thus acts as a natural anti-toxin. In addition, the bile contains combinations of stearine with gelatine and with carbonate and sulphate of sodium, which theoretical chemists believe are twin compounds of glycocholate and taurocholate. These fatty compounds depend upon stearine partly oxidized, that is deprived of a certain number of atoms of hydrogen.

As the compounds of fatty acids with ammoniacal blood gelatine and sodium carbonate, the ingredients of the bile also, develop into a peculiar soap. In the economy of the body the bile acts as a soap. When it is discharged into the duodenum, it changes the fats into so fine an emulsion (chyle) that the microscopically fine drops of fat may be drawn into the orifices of the lymph canals and conveyed to the circulatory system, and the cleavage products of albumen produced by gastric digestion, the peptones (leucin and tyrosin) are carried along with them for the renewal of tissue cells consumed in respiration.

If a soda soap is requisite for the purpose just stated, it follows that soda in the food is essential, as otherwise the supply of soda in the blood albumen cannot be renewed, and the bile cannot get its necessary supply of soda from blood albumen devoid of soda. Consequently, the entire nutritive process is dependent upon bile, and the bile cannot properly perform its function if denied soda.

In addition to carbonates of sodium, especially the hydrocarbonate known as glycolate, the bile apparently contains ammonium sulphate combined with hydrocarbon (taurin); but this results from the transposition of sodium sulphate and gelatine. Gelatine contains six atoms of hydrocarbon joined with two of ammonium carbonate, a group which is separable by chemical action into five of carburetted hydrogen with ammonium carbonate (leucin or gelatine milk), $C_5 H_{10}$, CO_2, NH_3, and into one of carburetted hydrogen with ammonium carbonate (glycin or gelatine sugar), CH_2, CO_2, NH_3. This latter substance, gelatine sugar, is not produced in the liver, as it exists already in the blood gelatine. In an isolated condition it has the property, in virtue of its ammoniacal acids and its carbonic acid bases and, therefore, of both combined, its salts, of producing chemical fixation. This property is conveyed to the undivided blood gelatine in which the gelatine sugar is contained intramolecularly.

Since normal blood albumen is inconceivable without sulphur it is absolutely essential, in accordance with our knowledge of the constituents of the bile and their origin, that our nutriment should contain a sufficiency of sodium sulphate, if normal blood serum is to be produced. The use of pepsin for this purpose cannot serve nature's purpose, as it contains neither sodium carbonate nor sodium sulphate. Our blood must be given a fresh and sufficient supply of sodium carbonate and sodium sulphate via our food, if it is to produce normal bile and supply the requisites of normal nutrition.

It is erroneously held that sodium sulphate is simply a laxative, even Borner's "Royal Medical Calendar" so classifies it. Often it discharges this function, it is true, in concentrated solution (one to five). But it is an important ingredient of healthy blood albumen (one to one thousand), and in this proportion assists in the formation of normal bile.

The blood of the Caucasian race is found to contain about ten parts of salt to the thousand, and this proportion of salt denotes firm tissue material. If the quantity of salt in the blood is diminished, the bi-concave red blood cells swell to a spherical form from access of water and lose their ability to unite for the production of connective tissue. Moreover, to the extent salt in the blood cells is decreased the connective tissue and muscle and tendon substance absorb water and the tissues become spongy, especially in the kidneys, so that the thinned blood albumen seeps through (urea albumen).

Phosphate of potassium is the mineral basis of muscle tissue, phosphate of lime with a small amount of magnesium phosphate the basis of bones, and phosphate of ammonium the bases of nervous tissue. There is a sufficient quantity of phosphate in all healthy foods. When the milk fed to nurslings, however, is greatly thinned with water instead of firm muscle fibers and solid lymph glands we find loose and spongy tissues. This is a scrofulous condition.

In the formation of healthy bones and teeth, calcium fluoride is essential. It is insoluble in plain water, but is made soluble by the aid of the glycocoll in blood gelatine and changed into ammonium fluoride. It appears in this form in the cartilaginous matter of the eye lenses, and lack of calcium fluoride in the food results in the clouding of these lenses.

Silicic acid is not only indispensible to the growth of hair, but it forms a direct connection between blood and nerve tissues. It is found in birds eggs, both in the white and the yolk. It is a conservator of heat and electricity as it is a good insulator. It also possesses eminent antiseptic qualities. Its mere presence in the intestinal canal, even its simple passage through the canal; conserves the electrical activity of the intestinal nerves and thus influences the whole sympathetic nervous system.

This brief review, cursory as it is, of the function of the minerals in the renewal of substances undergoing tissue change, makes it clear that our daily food must contain a sufficient quantity of them if healthy metabolism is to be maintained.

Chemically considered the human body is one individual whole, its characteristic chemical basis being gelatine. Lieut. C.E. McDonald, U.S.A. Medical Corps, recognized this when he recently wrote: "The similarity of chemical compositions explains why, when any particular region falls a prey to chemical decomposition, others quickly become affected."

Oxygen gas is the medium through which chemical combustion is carried on in the body for the purpose of preparing materials to enter into its composition. The mineral salts already named not only form the solid basis of the various tissue but also serve as conductors or insulators of electricity in the body. The absence of one of them for a protracted period is sufficient to explain widespread degeneration in the system.

In view of the fact that these various minerals play an indispensable part in healthy metabolism it is imperative that a sufficiency of them should be supplied in proper proportion in our daily food. It is imperative, if we desire to retain or to restore health to the body.

These mineral elements are to be found in the first instance in the earth, but they are of no use to the body in that form. We cannot digest and assimilate inorganic matter no matter how finely it may be pulverized. But plants can assimilate them from the earth and organize them in such form as to make them easily assimilable by animals and man.

If the soil on which our food is produced is itself deficient in some of these elements, our food must also lack them. If, moreover, we cannot for any reason add the missing elements to the soil, we must supply them to the human system in the shape of prepared nutritive salts. It is preferable, of course, that our food should contain all of the elements necessary for the proper nourishment of the body.

Thus we are forced to return to consideration of the soil. It is an established fact that our fields were originally formed from decayed rock, and analysis shows that this primitive rock contains the same minerals as healthy blood. But if our agriculturists are taught that stable manure and three or four other things are all that is necessary for the fertilization of their fields, where shall the other minerals essential to human metabolism come from?

What a man is, largely depends upon what he eats. Hence man is very largely a product of the fields. When the soil is denuded of any of the elements essential to plant and animal life, it must be properly fertilized. Incomplete or improper fertilization can have but one result, to-wit, it will produce sickly vegetation, and this in turn must produce unhealthy cattle, and since man is dependent upon plant and animal life for his food a sickly race of human beings is the ultimate result.

Is not barrenness of the soil responsible for disease in potatoes, for San Jose scale, Phylloxera, and other similar phenomena. The fields are manured profusely, it is true, but the very chemical elements which are not only essential to the development of wholesome plant tissue but which would also enable the plant to protect itself against parasites, are not used. Every farmer has observed, for instance, that grass grown upon cow dung in pastures is not eaten by cows, oxen or sheep. The instinct of the animals is correct.

In using the term incomplete fertilization, I mean supplying only potash, phosphoric acid and nitrogen, and possibly lime and sulphur, when the soil is denuded of several other elements. No matter how rich a field may be made in these things if it lacks other elements healthy vegetation cannot be grown in it.

Improper fertilization is another matter. It may consist in dressing a field with nothing but stable manure, or of applying crude sulphur or brimstone instead of using calcium sulphate—plus the other lacking elements. The advocate of crude sulphur certainly does not know how truly criminal his advice is. It is not to be denied that at the outset sulphur will increase the crop yield. But in the end—what? The sulphur will dissolve all of the essential minerals in the soil, and in the course of four or five years they will all be leached out and it will be so barren that not even wild grass can be grown upon it. Improper fertilization may also consist of a dressing of carbonate of lime applied at the wrong time or in excessive quantity. The effect of this course will be equally as harmful, namely, the transformation of the nitrogenous material into free nitrogen which will ascend to heaven. Without nitrogen albumen cannot be formed, and without albumen the formation of vegetable and animal tissue is impossible.

Wholesome soil may, then, be defined thus: It is such ground as contains a sufficient supply of humus and nitrogen and all of the essential mineral components of organic tissue. The problem of fertilization, therefore, consists of supplying any or all of these elements in which the soil is deficient. The aim of fertilization, as a rule, is merely to increase crop production. But this may prove to be not merely shortsighted, it may turn out to be a social crime. It is criminal, indeed, as a great many diseases are directly traceable to incomplete and improper fertilization.

Let us face the effect of attempting to fertilize our fields with nothing more than stable manure, which, it is true, supplies phosphoric acid, potash and nitrogen. We know that phosphorus forms the foundation of nerves, and too much of it provokes nerve irritation in exact ratio to the deficiency of sulphur. There should be twice as many sulphuric salts as phosphoric salts in the blood, if it is to be normal and the nerves are to be steady. Foodstuffs from fields that have been fertilized in this manner must, of course, contain a superabundance of phosphoric salts and be deficient in sulphuric salts. Is it strange, then, that the present age presents a picture of restless, irritated nervous activity and thoughtless action?

We must return to the primitive rock and humbly learn the lesson it has for us, and upon this rock we must rear our science of fertilization and nutrition. This rock consisted of granite, porphyry, gneiss and basalt, and these are still found upon the earth in immense quantities in practically the same condition they were thousands of years ago. Both Justus von Liebig and Julius Hensel, as a matter of fact, advocated that this rock should be finely pulverized and used as a compost to assist in restoring and maintaining the original fertility of the soil and thus aid the development of healthy plant and animal life.

Indeed the instincts of both animals and human beings lead them under certain conditions right back to the rock and its lesson. Note the avidity with which hens confined in arid runs devoid of vegetation, worms, insects and small stones devour a compound of lime and ground bones and oyster shells. Observe a child whose ration is deficient in mineral elements eating egg shells, wall plaster, chalk and other earthy substances. What do these things mean? Nothing more than this: both chicken and child express a natural craving for the essential elements to build bone and form the basis for the tissue.

I have discussed the important part the minerals play in both the vegetable and animal kingdoms for the purpose of laying stress upon our great need of more of them in our daily diet, and I may add that this is equally as true in the case of those we call healthy as of those who are diseased. No matter how carefully the diet may be regulated as regards the quantity of protein and carbohydrates and fats and the ratio between them, healthy metabolism is impossible without a sufficiency of the essential minerals.

II.

How can we perform this imperative duty to mankind?

The solution of the problem of supplying these essential minerals demands that our soil shall be properly fertilized for the growing of wholesome vegetables and fruits and our cattle properly fed with a ration rich in mineral content. Thus the food which we eat will contain all of the elements necessary to the growth and maintenance of our bodies in a state of health.

In the course of my effort to show why it is imperative that we pay greater heed to the mineral content of our foodstuffs, and why it is imperative that we enrich that content, I have shown basically how that end is to be attained.

In conclusion I will cite the result of a series of experiments in applying the principles of physiological chemistry to poultry, and I may say that it took me twelve years to find the breed which would most readily lend itself to my purpose. I experimented with 250 varieties of hens before I found the one most amenable to my method of feeding and breeding.

While living at Needham, Massachusetts, I made a thorough test of my principles with the selected variety of hens. They were not only fed a ration properly balanced for protein, carbohydrates and fat, but I gave them a liberal supply of properly prepared mineral salts. I used three different mixtures of feed, made up in 100 pound lots, in which the proportion of albumen ranged from 13.50 to 18.00 pounds; of fat from 4.00 to 5.00 pounds; of carbohydrates from 41 to 44 pounds; and actual nutritive salts from 4.50 to 5.00 pounds. The respective ratios being: 1:4, 1:3.5 and 1:3

It is not necessary to enter into discussion of the details of the feeding method and the variation in the daily handling of the hens. The result of this experiment, however, was completely satisfactory, as the eggs produced by those hens not only contained a startling increase in the quantity of mineral salts, but their fertility was far greater than that of hens handled in the usual manner. The increase of fertility in itself is, it seems to me, the best proof of the soundness of my theoretical premises.

Some of the results of this experiment were published in the Reliable Poultry Journal in 1905, and Dr. Woods offered confirmatory evidence of the soundness of my conclusions two years later, after he had himself experimented along the same line.

I will cite just one fact revealed by that experiment, namely, that whereas 100 grams of dried egg yolk ordinarily contains only from 10 to 20 milligram of iron the eggs of those hens yielded from 30 to 80 milligrams. And all of the minerals were increased from 10 to 25 per cent or more.

The method of applying the principles of physiological chemistry to the enriching of the mineral content of our foodstuffs evolved by me is, with due recognition of the difference between the vegetable and animal kingdoms, equally applicable in the raising of all our foodstuffs with an augmented mineral content. I will adduce just one result of my work in the handling of small fruit: on the average, 100 grams of dried strawberries will yield 8.6 to 9.3 milligrams of iron, but strawberries raised by me yield from 30 to 40 milligrams per 100 grams.

In view of the facts with regard to the function of these minerals, it is indisputably true that a ration is physiologically inefficient if it does not contain a sufficiency of them in proper proportion. Moreover, this is trebly true in the case of those whose constitution has been weakened by loss of blood from rounds, by shell shock and trench fever, and of those here at home whose nerve tissue has been degenerated and whose blood has been weakened by anxiety and the strain of unwonted manual labor. The last consideration applies with especial force to the multitudes of women who have entered industry as manual laborers. What kind of offspring can we expect from these people whose plasma is thus degenerated? The children are the citizens of the future, and even before they are born we must plan for their health.

What could be more effective in treating the anaemic condition of wounded and crippled boys, and in treating the same condition in women industrial workers, than haemoglobin eggs?

What could be more efficacious in treating conditions arising from shell shock, from bad wounds and operations thereon, and neurasthenia in general, than an abundance of lecithin (which, as you know, dear doctor, is made from the yolk of the egg)?

What could be more successfully used in treating conditions arising from shattered bones and from operations for the removal of bone tissue than calcareous eggs in connection with a ration perfectly balanced as regards all of the other essential elements.

For the regeneration of the blood and bone and nerve tissue of these victims of war, something more than a sufficiency of nutritive food, as that term is commonly used, is needed, and something more than medicine is needed!

I am the last person in the world to deny that wonderful progress is made in surgery every day, and the last to fail to applaud its successful efforts, but you know quite as well as I do that in 90 out of 100 cases recovery involves exhaustion of the patient's reserve energy. Moreover, when the reserve energy has already been drawn upon almost to the point of exhaustion, no matter how successful the operation may be the recovery of the patient is a very doubtful quantity. The first requisite in all surgical cases, as also in all anaemic and neurasthenic cases, is to restore metabolism to its normal condition and thus help the patient to regain his reserve energy in order to prevent the collapse of the whole fabric.

It is indubitably true that healthy metabolism and the restoration of reserve energy depends upon the organism being given the requisite quantity of the sixteen essential elements of organic life in easily digestible and assimilable form, and I am asking for the opportunity to demonstrate how foods extremely rich in these elements may be produced and used to aid nature. I have not entered into a full discussion of the various aspects of my method of accomplishing that, but have confined myself to consideration of the basic principles underlying it. Neither have I attempted to show how these different minerals will serve as regenerative agents in different dysaemic conditions. I am prepared to discuss the matter from both of these viewpoints, however, and, more than that, I am ready to practically demonstrate the soundness of my theories, when given an opportunity under proper conditions to do so.

—Sapienti sat—

FINIS.

NUTRITIVE COMPOSITIONS.

The sixteen substances,—nutritive cell foods,—of which all of the tissues of the body are composed are: carbon, oxygen, hydrogen, nitrogen, potassium, soda, lime, magnesia, iron, manganese, phosphor, sulphur, silica, chlorine, fluorine and iodine.

My nutritive compositions consist of these same sixteen nutritive salts, each composition mixed in the same proportion as they are found in the healthy tissue for the regeneration of which they are prescribed.

Since in various diseases not only one but several tissues are affected, it must be decided individually in each case whether only one, or several, of the nutritive compositions will require to be taken, and in what proportion.

In accordance with the system of the twelve tissues of the body, the twelve nutritive compositions, commonly known as "DECH-MANNA" Compositions, are the following:

No. 1. Plasmogen   Bloodplasma-Producer.

No. 2. Lymphogen   Lymph-Cell-Producer.

No. 3. Neurogen   Nerve-cell-Producer.

No. 4. Osseogen   Bone-cell-Producer.

No. 5. Muscogen   Muscle-cell-Producer.

No. 6. Mucogen   Mucous membrane-cell-Producer.

No. 7. Dento-Ophthogen   Tooth and Eye-cell-Producer.

No. 8. Capillogen   Hair-cell-Producer.

No. 9. Dermogen   Skin-cell-Producer.

No. 10. Gelatinogen   Gelatigenous-cell-Producer.

No. 11. Cartilogen   Cartilage-cell-Producer.

No. 12. Eubiogen   Healthy body-cell-Producer.

In addition to these I use only a few specialities in certain cases of disease, viz.:

A. Oxygenator   A radium emanation for the bath.

B. Eubiogen Liquid   Same as No. 12, but liquid form.

C. Tonogen   A stimulating tonic.

D. Tea. Diabetic, Dechmann

E. Tea. Laxagen, after Kneipp

F. Salve. Lenicet, after Dr. Reiss

G. Massage Emulsion, Dechmann

H. Propionic acid for steam atomizer

I. Oxygen Powder, after Hensel

J. Anti-Phosphate, Dechmann

(These specialities are used only in certain individual cases, according to prescription).

NUTRITIVE COMPOSITIONS.

In discussing the various preparations of Dech-Manna-Diet, I refrain from detailed prescription and analysis. My intention is to explain them in such a way that it may become apparent to everyone that they are rational remedies for every properly diagnosed constitutional disease. If I should do more than this, it would be simply placing a premium upon unscrupulous imitations. For the present therefore, I prefer to have the remedies prepared exclusively by accredited and absolutely reliable chemists of first class local standing, in order that I may myself assume the entire responsibility. In cases of illness, however, it is always necessary to consult a biological-hygienic physician. The Dech-Manna-Diet remedies, for the time being, will always be obtainable on application to myself, to be administered in accordance with such medical directions. I trust that very shortly when official and general recognition will permit, I shall be enabled to entrust the detailed prescriptions to a wider circle of practising physicians and chemists.

In order to illustrate how necessary it is to abstain from more detailed description of my remedies, I will cite but one of several incidents which happened to me in course of practice.

In the year 1905, I wrote a number of articles for the "Reliable Poultry Journal" on the scientific feeding of chickens, and gave, amongst other tables, two food-formulas of the mineral contents of *chicken food rations*. (Both formulas were copyrighted). I gave the same gratis, for private personal use. A certain "Chicken Specialist" from the Orange River Colony, South Africa, first wrote a glowing article upon the wonderful success he had secured with my prescriptions. Not satisfied with this, however, he conceived a brilliant idea of great possibilities of future income to be derived therefrom. He left South Africa and came to America, the country of unlimited possibilities, and settled in Los Angeles, California, where he floated a company, which sells my copyrighted prescriptions for poultry feeding, to all and sundry as specifics for all possible and impossible ailments. This ambitious gentleman even went so far as to offer my labouriously earned discoveries to the United States Government. — But further comment is unnecessary!

This is but one of numerous instances of the kind some of which are embodied in a little treatise I have published, free to my friends, entitled "A Message to the Thinker."

Patients sometimes ask me what my methods have in common with "Schuessler's Tissue Remedies."

I answer: Nothing—absolutely nothing, as the explanation will show.

Schuessler's therapy claims that the minerals are needful to build up the system; but he only uses one trillionth part of a gram and *imagines* that the remainder is to be found in the food. Now anybody with a fair understanding can easily figure that if a patient of middle age eventually loses through disease about 200 grams of lime, it is simply a farce to claim that the above dose of $1/100,000,000,000$ of a gram (which is the homeopathic dose of Schuessler), will cure or replace the lime which was lost.

There are other equally erroneous pretentions in Schuessler's therapy which are really too silly to go into in detail. Time and space are too valuable to squander on any such puerile hypothesis.

DECH-MANNA-DIET.

MENTOR TO PRESCRIPTIONS.

It may be well to preface this summary of prescriptions with the following explanatory remarks; namely,

(1) That while my compositions are usually taken in the form of powders, they may be taken in the form of capsules or tablets, in which case the dose given is always exact.

They may also be mixed with Eubiogen or various kinds of food, except where this is strictly forbidden by the physician.

Such mixtures cannot be harmful, since they consist of components from which our body-cells are constructed. They may be taken either singly, or as compounds.

(2) As regards the matter of quantities:—

Whenever one-fourth teaspoonful is mentioned, the meaning is that one-fourth of a *heaping* teaspoonful be taken.

Whenever a *level* one-fourth teaspoonful is meant, as in the case of plasmogen, it is because the basic remedy is heavier and, therefore, the smaller quantity renders an equal amount in weight.

Every dose mentioned herein contains the exact amount of the necessary constituents, and the harmonious system of dosage which I have worked out, consists of reducing every compound dosage to one gram, which weight is equal to about one quarter teaspoonful of the regular preparation, made lighter and fluffier through trituration with milk-sugar.

This trituration is a manual process and requires some three hours steady and continuous rubbing of the ingredients with pestle and mortar, for each separate composition.

All my compositions should be kept in a dry and cool place. It is best to put them into wide-mouthed bottles with glass stoppers, as they are all hygroscopic, that is, sensitive to moisture.

DECH-MANNA COMPOSITION No. 1.
PLASMOGEN (PLASMA PRODUCER.)

Plasmogen—Blood-plasma producer. (The red and white blood-corpuscles are produced by using Eubiogen, XII).

(a). Blood-plasma, is the habitat of the red and white blood-corpuscles.

It can be readily understood that the more sanitary a place, the better will be the condition of those who live in it. Therefore, the plasma, (blood-plasma), must first be made as perfect as possible in accordance with the teachings of science and especially of biology,—a theory which my own experience has proved to be correct.

No matter how perfect the red or white corpuscles may be, if they live in diseased blood-plasma, they cannot perform their functions properly and, as a consequence, the resistant power of the system is crippled.

(b). Plasmogen contains all the constituents in the proportions in which they should be contained in perfect plasma.

The Law of the Minimum teaches that if one of the ingredients is lacking in the food, the cells *must* become diseased. This the great Justus v. Liebig emphasized when he said: "If the most minute component is lacking, the rest cannot perform their functions." Taken as directed, the plasmogen is also in its natural dosage.

It was only after years of ardent study that I was enabled to produce this composition in the perfect form in which it is furnished today.

Since the plasmogen contains all the salts necessary to keep the blood in perfect harmony, the circulation as well as the resistant power will be maintained, the heart relieved, the fighting capacity of the white corpuscles strengthened, and therefore the power of disease very greatly reduced.

(c). In all cases of constitutional disease, plasmogen is used to bring about a proper regeneration and preservation of the blood-cells. In all cases of acute, febrile diseases its purpose is to bring about a proper circulation and fluid condition of the blood-cells.

The most wonderful results will accrue through the use of plasmogen in *all acute* febrile cases, particularly in the case of children; also by using the same as directed in individual cases of constitutional diseases. It is indispensable in producing bactericide blood, which is necessary to regenerate the body-cells. Therefore, I recommend It in *all* Regenerative Treatments.

How many thousands of children may be saved by this single remedy alone only the biologist who has studied life according to the teachings of nature's laws, is able to appreciate today. It will take some time before the general medical practitioner will realize the truth of this statement, because the old-school medicine does not teach these facts.

Therefore it is the duty of every thoughtful mother to prevent harm to her children resulting from the drugs they favour. All anti-febrile chemicals are rank poisons and contrary to nature's way. *Only by producing a higher temperature is nature able to throw off impurities*; but in many cases this becomes dangerous, because so very few know how to avoid an over-taxation of nature's strength. Instead of assisting nature by keeping the head cool, the feet warm and the bowels and pores open, the anxious mothers will wrap their babies up nicely, give them some patent or other obnoxious medicine, and really kill nature's efforts by means of narcotics and other poisons. Results are always fatal. The mother must learn to use correct, harmless remedies and to follow the instructions given nearly 3000 years ago by the wise Hippocrates, the "Father of Medicine," who warned every medical practitioner with these words: "Nil nocere." (Never do harm).

(d). *Dose*: In acute cases, that is to say, in emergency cases where the patient, for instance a child, has developed a high temperature, and the doctor has not as yet diagnosed any special form of disease, or has been unable to do so because the time of incubation of the germ has not passed, give the patient a dose of plasmogen, that is, one gram, or as much as will lie on a ten-cent piece, or one-fourth of a level teaspoonful. Dissolve it in one-half tumbler of water, (or milk if prescribed), and let the patient drink it slowly at intervals, as seems necessary.

In ordinary cases individual directions should be followed.

DECH-MANNA COMPOSITION No. II.
LYMPHOGEN (LYMPH CELL PRODUCER.)

(a). In nearly every tissue and organ of the body there is a marvelous network of vessels, called the lymphatics. These are busily at work taking up and making over waste fluids or surplus materials derived from the blood and tissues generally. The lymphatics seem to spring from the parts in which they are found, like the rootlets of a plant in the soil. They carry a turbid, slightly yellowish fluid, called lymph, very much like blood without the red corpuscles. The lymph is carried to the lymphatic glands where it undergoes certain changes to fit it for entering the blood.

It is a fact that very few doctors know, that the whole nervous system can only be fed by the lymph, whose central station is the so-called ductus thoracicus (thoracic duct), in the upper region of the chest. As there is no pulsation or magnetism connected with the same, the body must lie down and rest at night. Then and only then is the system enabled to feed all the nerve centers, especially through the influence of the sympathetic nerve system, which may be said to work in the form of a relay station, through its inherent power from the very beginning. Therefore, it becomes quite a task to regenerate a broken-down nervous system, for those practitioners who are not familiar with physiological chemistry—that is, life chemistry, which teaches the composition of the tissues. The law of chemotaxis will explain it. The lymphatic system also plays a great part in constitutional diseases of the blood. Every degeneration of the blood cells, or dysaemia, is influenced more or less by the perfect condition of the lymphatic fluid. All cachectic or morbid nutrition conditions are due to imperfect lymph.

(b). Lymphogen contains all the organic minerals in the same proportion in which they are contained in perfect lymph, and if taken as directed, will always restore the lymphatic system and allow it to perform its important function.

(c). The great importance of perfect lymph will be understood from the previous remarks, especially those pertaining to the feeding of the whole nervous system. If the lymphatic system is impeded by underfeeding or inanition of the nerve-cells, how can any one with common sense expect such a system to be in perfect working order and harmony? This applies particularly to those constitutional diseases where the lymphatic system and the lymph itself are degenerating through causes due to heredity, predisposition or acquisition of such conditions.

(d). *Dose*: Twice daily I gram or one-fourth heaping teaspoonful or, if in tablet form, I tablet, dry or with a little water or in foodstuffs; to be taken at 10 a.m. and 4 p.m. or as specially directed.

DECH-MANNA COMPOSITION No. III.
NEUROGEN (NERVE CELL PRODUCER).

(a). The nerves are the cord-like structures which convey impulses from one part of the body to another.

The tremendous importance of their absolute health is obvious, since the co-operation of all parts of the human body depends upon it, while, on the other hand, their very delicate structure exposes them to numerous and easily acquired forms of disease.

(b). This composition contains all the constituents required to generate nerve tissue. The most important and expensive is lecithin. Pure lecithin, the kind I use, is made from the yolks of fresh eggs. In this composition I supply nutritive cell-food for generating lecithin in exactly the same form in which it is found in a healthy, perfect nerve-cell. It is absolutely digestible and assimilable, and is triturated with the finest milk sugar.

(c). All morbid conditions caused by imperfect nerve-cells can be regenerated through this composition as long as there is some foundation left on which to work.

Under an endless variety of names—as a matter of fact, a big book would not be sufficient to describe all so-called "nervous diseases"—it can be readily seen in what a brainless way some "nerve specialists" classify patients of this kind. Not knowing the constituents of the nerve-cells, they still attempt to prescribe for neurasthenic patients. The results are in accordance with such travesty of treatment. The increase in the number of Insane Asylums gives, or should give, a true picture of existing conditions. What is needed is a little more knowledge of physiological chemistry, but as it is too much to expect of the ordinary so-called "nerve specialist" to be familiar with this science, we must per force be content with the prevailing condition, that is, a condition characterized by ignorance of the most vital laws of being.

But what reasonable ground of complaint, let me ask, have the people, themselves, in this matter?

Of the appalling results of the prevailing medical system, recognized as it is by the law of the land and supported and virtually endorsed by the people's own will and prejudices, they themselves, though well aware, are yet complacent. But, mark it well, not until independent medicine shall be accorded reasonable recognition, a fair field and general fair play, and the chance afforded to science outside the "orthodox" medical clique to inaugurate some drastic measures of urgently needed reform, not until then will it be possible to alter this disastrous state of affairs—not until then will matters become less unbearable to the individual and less discreditable to every one concerned. *We can cure disease only by removing its cause; this is my maxim and it is true for all time.*

Much of neurasthenia is due to the degenerate times in which we are now living. Causes must be removed in every line of life, political, social, and economical, before normal physical and mental conditions can be restored. Then neurasthenia, in all its forms, will be a disease of the past, but not before—not withstanding the frequent alleged discoveries of serums and antidotes of wonder-working properties so triumphantly heralded from the "Halls of Science."

(d). *Dose*: Twice daily, 1 gram or one-fourth heaping teaspoonful or, it in tablet form, 1 tablet, dry or with a little water or in food-stuffs; to be taken at 10 a.m. and 4 p.m. or as specially directed.

DECH-MANNA COMPOSITION No. IV.
OSSEOGEN (BONE CELL PRODUCER).

(a). If I tell you that it takes seven different compositions of organic lime to make perfect bones, some people, even very learned ones, may doubt my word. But biology and physiological chemistry teach that this is so—and prove it. If this composition were lacking in a certain quantity of organic magnesia, the bones would grow hard and brittle. It is the magnesia that turns the tissue into perfect, elastic form.

(b). Osseogen is the composition the constituents of which are necessary to generate perfect bone tissue. How many troubles could easily be prevented by using this cell-food in time!

(c). This composition becomes an absolute essential in all cases of imperfect bone structure, such as rachitis, or rickets, constitutional disease of children, osteomalacia, tuberculosis of the bones, deformity of bone structure, such as curvature of the spine, etc.

Softening of the bones, known as osteomalacia, curvature of the spine, rachitis and many other terrible conditions of disease would not be known to humanity if proper precaution were taken in time.

Hundreds of patients are today cured by my method of supplying this lacking constituent in a form assimilable to even the smallest infant.

Lime-water and such imaginary substitutes are pure nonsense, as must surely be apparent to even the simplest layman when they consider for a moment that it takes seven different lime compositions in order to supply the necessary lime for generating bone tissue. Is it necessary to say more to convince even a dogmatist? How indispensable osseogen becomes may be realized when people begin to know enough about themselves to realize that our bone structure must be "fireproof" in order to last for the normal span of human life!

(d). *Dose*: Once or twice daily, according to the individual case. 1 gram will be sufficient for a proper dose. As stated before, one-fourth of a heaping teaspoonful is equal to a gram.

It may be that in a short while I shall be able to supply all these compositions in tablet form in their respective doses. Then medication will become still more simple. This composition may also be taken in food or a little water.

DECH-MANNA COMPOSITION No. V.
MUSCOGEN (MUSCLE CELL PRODUCER).

(a). The term muscle signifies every organ of the human body which, by contraction, produces the movements of the organism. Muscles are of the greatest variety and strength, but all consist of the same chemical elements, and can be regenerated in case of disease, like every other organ, by feeding the patient with the chemical substances which the muscle cells require.

(b). Into this composition I have introduced the components necessary for muscle tissue.

The basis of this form of cell-food is potassium phosphate. It will regenerate all muscular tissue when used as directed. All minerals contained therein are organized and in a perfectly digestible and assimilable form. Even an infant can easily digest it. It will prevent all decompositions of the muscular system and regenerate the cells as long as any basis for life is left.

(c). As it is impossible for even the healthiest system to build up new tissue without the necessary proportion of albumen, it becomes very important to use the right proportion and form of this component. Therefore, all patients who are in need of this special tissue builder, must at the same time take the main composition, Eubiogen (life producer). Under No. XII, I will endeavor to give the reader some little idea of its properties, and describe its marvelous regenerating powers.

(d). *Dose*: 1 gram, or one-fourth of a heaping teaspoonful once or twice daily will be sufficient. It may have to be taken for 3, 6, 9 or 12 months, and even longer. Everything depends upon the cause of the degeneration of the muscle tissue.

DECH-MANNA COMPOSITION No. VI.
MUCOGEN (MUCOUS MEMBRANE CELL PRODUCER).

(a). The entire intestines, the stomach, all cavities, organs, openings of the body, the genital and urinary tracts, etc., are lined with mucous membrane, which must always be kept in a normal and healthy condition, otherwise the functions of metabolism and procreation of the organism cannot be carried on in safety and health.

(b). Mucogen consists of all the constituents necessary for the building up of the peculiarly tender tissue called mucous membrane. These constituents are absolutely indispensible, and nature must be supplied with them if disease of the mucous membrane is to be healed by removing its cause.

(c). The tenderness of this tissue is obvious, and experience has shown how much it is exposed to changes in its normal condition, how easily an increase or decrease in its main functions is brought about. While this increase or decrease in many instances is a natural fight of nature against the intrusion of opposing elements into the body, it frequently assumes dimensions that are most unpleasant and seriously impair the health, such as catarrhal conditions, all of which are due to poor or degenerated cells of this tissue.

The frequent occurence of this form of disease shows the importance of always supplying the cells of this tissue with the substances that keep them in health, or if need be, will regenerate them.

(d). *Dose*: 1 gram or one-fourth of a heaping teaspoonful once or twice daily will be found sufficient to supply the requirements.

In some instances this composition, as well as others, may be mixed with the main composition Eubiogen, in order that the patient may digest it more readily, especially in the case of a child.

Special directions must always be followed closely.

DECH-MANNA COMPOSITION No. VII.

DENTO AND OPHTHOGEN (TOOTH AND EYE CELL PRODUCER).

This refers to the enamel of the teeth and the crystalline lens of the eye.

(a). Two special tissues of the human body, the close connection between which has been observed and recognized but very little, contain a predominant quantity of fluoride of lime, and consequently may be placed under one heading in this system, although the basis for the fluorate of the teeth is calcium, while the basis of the crystalline lens of the eye is gelatine.

(b). I have composed this cell-food, containing the necessary fluoride of lime, in this particular way in order to avoid too much specialization. From long years of practical experience I have found that the special cells of each tissue will take up only those constituents which they need for the construction of their respective tissue, as taught by the law of chemotaxis.

(c). Composition No. VII will be prescribed in case of tooth and eye troubles. Any observant student of human nature will have noticed that in severe cases of degeneration (as for instance, diabetes) not only one of these two tissues mentioned above is affected, (as the decaying and falling out of the teeth), but in most cases also the other (as cataract of the eye). Some doctors of course may ask what in the world the tooth has to do with the eye. But, alas! they have yet much to learn. The two are not so distinct from each other when one understands. I fear that later on, when this method, which is the only true and natural one, comes into practice, everything will be specialized to such an extent that the real science of it will become so complicated that the proverb—"Veritatis simplex oratio est"—(The language of truth is simple)—will become entirely obsolete.

It is my endeavor to state the pure unvarnished truth, and in terms as simple as possible; that is my mission.

(d). *Dose*: One gram or one-fourth of a heaping teaspoonful, or one tablet in a little water or milk, once a day will be sufficient except in very severe cases of degenerated tissue.

DECH-MANNA COMPOSITION No. VIII.

CAPILLOGEN (HAIR CELL PRODUCER).

(a). The hair is built of a number of elements not contained in other tissues of the body, and which must be supplied in order to keep the hair in good health and prevent it from falling out.

(b). Capillogen contains all the necessary constituents in proper proportion required by perfect hair tissue.

(c). The main disease of the hair, responsible for this falling out, may be due, to two different causes. It may be due to the quality of the hair, or to the condition of the nutritive soil of that part of the skin where hair is wont to grow. If the loss of hair is due to the first cause, its regeneration, through Dech-Manna Composition No. VIII, naturally gives rise to the hope that the lost hair may be replaced, if the process of regeneration is not begun too late, as is usually the case.

My composition, however, is not a "hair restorer."

As a great many of my readers may know, and some of them to their sorrow, all so-called hair restorers on the market are failures—although perhaps not so to the manufacturer or clever salesman.

My composition will prevent the hair tissues from degeneration. Thus baldness, which might otherwise have occurred in a larger or smaller degree, may be prevented.

In the case of the disability of the skin to retain the hair, which may occur after forms of febrile disease, such as typhoid fever, or if children show little promise of growing nice hair, the composition will prove very useful in combination with Dech-Manna Composition No. XII, Eubiogen, which restores the original strength of the whole body, while hair regenerated by the blood through capillogen has a better chance of growing and remaining in the regenerated soil.

(d). *Dose*: One gram or one-fourth of a heaping teaspoonful, or one tablet in a little water or milk, once a day. It is imperative to follow directions implicitly.

DECH-MANNA COMPOSITION No. IX.
DERMOGEN (SKIN CELL PRODUCER).

(a). The skin, like all other tissues of the body, is made up of different constituent elements. While its disease appears on the outside, it is built up, like all other parts of the human organism, from within and through the blood only. The elements necessary for regenerating the skin and keeping it in a healthy condition must, therefore, also be supplied to the body from within, in the form of nutriment, as otherwise, though we might suppress and eliminate the symptoms, the disease would still remain.

(b). Dermogen, skin producer, contains all the constituent elements which a healthy skin tissue requires.

(c). The skin, being exposed to all external influences, discloses the symptoms of all forms of skin disease, the names of which are legion.

The skin specialist termed "dermatologist" is another production which flourishes — more or less — upon the ignorance of the public. The patient, alas, is less fortunate. He tries one after another until disgusted he sometimes resorts to special diet. Sometimes this may help, if he choose a certain kind of vegetable diet, and especially if the vegetables are such as contain a great deal of silica; for silica is the mineral basis of skin tissue. Full details of this are to be found in my analysis of foodstuffs given in the chart at the end of volume No. I of my work, "Regeneration."

(d). *Dose*: One gram or one-fourth of a heaping teaspoonful of dermogen in a little water or milk once a day until regeneration of the skin is fairly started. Reduce the dose gradually until complete recovery has been accomplished.

DECH-MANNA COMPOSITION No. X.
GELATINOGEN (GELATIGENOUS TISSUE PRODUCER).

(a). All blood and lymphatic vessels, the alveoli of the lungs, all tendons and cords in the entire system, the bowel tract, including the stomach, the bladder, and in fact every organ or tissue which has the function of expanding and contracting, must be of healthy gelatigenous (rubber-like) tissue; otherwise it cannot perform its functions in the system and must degenerate.

(b). Gelatinogen contains the constituent elements of gelatine, which it carries, through the blood, to the parts of the body where it is needed to rebuild degenerated gelatigenous tissue.

(c). While there are not many special forms of disease of the gelatigenous tissues, many diseased conditions are more or less connected with its degeneration. In fact, every layman should be able to judge the importance of perfect gelatigenous tissue. But how many human beings ever think of such things. Yet they know very well that a poor rubber tire on an automobile will not last very long or stand much strain; for the fact appeals to the pocket book—and that degenerates.

It is well to learn the truth before too late and give, to the rising generation at least, the chance to which they are surely entitled:—A good healthy body.

(d). *Dose*: Twice daily, 1 gram or one-fourth of a heaping tea-spoonful, or one tablet, at 10 a.m. and 4 p.m., or as individually prescribed, in a little water, milk or other foodstuffs, to be taken for a certain length of time.

DECH-MANNA COMPOSITION No. XI
CARTILOGEN (CARTILAGE PRODUCER).

(a). Every bone in the human system must be covered with carti-lage at its ends so as to prevent self-destruction through friction, especially in the joints.

(b). Cartilogen consists of all the necessary constituents of this important material, and under certain circumstances it must be introduced in this concentrated form, as for instance when the gen-eral diet is unable to counteract the influences of disease which tends to degenerate the cartilage and subjects the body to the great suffering which the absence of cartilage invariably produces.

(c). Cartilage keeps all the joints in working order and must be regenerated constantly.

As soon as the blood and lymph no longer contain the proper, necessary constituents for the rebuilding of cartilage tissue, the consequence is degeneration of this tissue.

It is obvious then that the presence of proper cartilage constituents in the blood is of the greatest importance to the regenerating forces in the human body. Our foodstuffs, therefore, must contain the material in a digestible, assimilable form, thus to prevent inanition of the cells, otherwise degeneration of the cartilage tissue must follow.

(d). *Dose*: One gram or one-fourth of a heaping teaspoonful twice a day for a certain period, depending on the condition of the patient. This may be taken in the same manner as previously described.

DECH-MANNA COMPOSITION No. XII.
EUBIOGEN (HEALTHY LIFE PRODUCER). (ALSO TERMED "POSITIVE COMPOSITION").

(a). While all other compositions contain *special* elements for the rebuilding of *special* tissues through regeneration of *special* cells, Eubiogen contains a combination of all the important elements in the most concentrated form. I was fortunate enough, after years of experimenting with plants and animal life, to concentrate the solid constituents of the human body *ten* fold. The full import of this achievement few can realize, but those who know what it means in time and study. The effect of this composition is felt simultaneously in all the vital tissues of the body, and since the co-operation of all these tissues is what we call "life," I feel there is no name more fitting for this product than the one I have selected, namely, "Eubiogen," or "Healthy Life Producer." I maintain that it is the most scientific composition discovered since the time of Hippocrates and the following is its analysis:

It has at all times been an ideal aim of mankind to produce a species of food that would combine a minimum of quantity with a maximum of quality, and philosophers and scientists have dreamed of a time when the day's portion of foodstuffs would be concentrated in one small pill. The biologist cannot accept this theory.

While Greek mythology seemed to symbolize a similar idea; namely, of one concentrated food-substance combining all nutritive elements, as represented in their "Ambrosia," the food of the Gods.

Yet the gods and goddesses were permitted to partake of it only at solemn assemblies when all sat at the table of Zeus and enjoyed their food and drank its liquid counterpart, termed "nectar."

This symbolism represented Ambrosia and Nectar as the highest climax of food; just as the Greek gods stood for the climax of various human qualities, in each case attributed to one single personality.

The Greeks knew well that the human body requires a variety of food in order to remain healthy. It is an echo of the same thought expressed in the Bible when the Jews are given the "Manna" only in the utmost emergency. The Bible also advocates a considerable variety of food, regarding which the Old Testament lays down the most careful and explicit regulations.

In praising "Ambrosia" as the climax of food-substances, Greek mythology attributed to it the power not only of regeneration, but of procreation. For the reproduction of healthy human life in its offspring, was to them just as sacred and important a preoccupation as it was natural, to ensure the survival of the race; and to secure to all the food that would assist in this, their highest and most worthy aim, seemed to them a manifest duty which, at the present day, prudish "morality" either practically ignores or modestly pretends to neglect. Healthy food, generally speaking, will do much towards ensuring healthy offspring.

But the times of extreme leisure, as enjoyed by the ancient Greeks, are long past and a more exacting age makes its more strenuous demands upon the human tissues, and in innumerable cases causes them to deteriorate more rapidly than they can be regenerated and restored to their original vigor by even the healthiest food.

Hence I have felt justified, in considering the best interests of the race—present and future—in devoting the crowning effort of my long scientific career to the production of modern biological remedies such as would be felt in the reproductive powers of the people—a consideration concerning which the old-time, prudish reticence is a foolish figment rapidly passing away.

Now, as regards myself and my great work. Surely to boast a little is but human. The man who puts his very best efforts into an ideal, and having achieved it, has not striven to reap the fruits thereof for selfish gain, but year by year, has perfected that work until the tests have finally permitted him to cry: "Eureka"—it is accomplished beyond dispute,—that man has the right to overstep the conventional rule which forbids self-praise. While in other work accomplished I see but the links of an uncompleted chain, the synthesis of Eubiogen, I feel to be one of those so rare occasions in human life, when a tested accomplishment allows and even demands a somewhat different treatment. And so I have the courage to speak as follows in eulogy of my own production:

This product is my masterpiece. I am proud of it. Nothing like it in efficiency has ever before been given to the world. In the fullest sense of the word, it is in food value the most perfect concentration that science and research have ever evolved. It is the result of the quest of 30 years and should make its finder famous. Hundreds of men of mark have each one given to mankind some noble token of their genius; but of such gifts not one possessed the concentrated virtues, the materialized knowledge of "Eubiogen." This, to unsympathetic ears, may sound like vain, exaggerated vapouring;—but it is not so. *It is the truth*. It is impossible to describe the real value of its properties within a limited space. Sufferers in their thousands will yet live to be grateful for the benefits derived from it, and the full and positive knowledge of its excellence makes it the more difficult to describe in a few weak words. An abler pen than mine would fail to do it justice.

In sentimental somnolence I sometimes dream how, perhaps, in the days to come, another hand may write in glowing terms the faithful history of "Eubiogen" and say kind feeling words and fair of the hard worked lone scientist who gave its healing virtues to mankind, terming it—he too perhaps—the stereotyped "Ambrosia," the diet of the Olympian gods; but for myself, it is all I ask to know that it has served the appointed end to which my energy has aimed,— that it has proved a food instinct with healing and comfort to my kind—a staunch support and refuge for the overwrought sinews of humanity. May such be my guerdon of reward for the long years of thought and toil and—I shall rest content.

(b). Eubiogen contains the best and purest ingredients science and experience can produce today. It is the most delicate and at the same time the most digestible and assimilable cell-food obtainable.

Many great names since the time of Hippocrates have figured in the list of those who shared with me the ambitious hope to give mankind some wonder-working remedy — Metschnikoff, Voit, Koenig, Biedert, Rubner, Gruber, Kussmaul, Bischoff, Teschemacher, Hirschfeld, Boemer, Wintgen, Virchow, Hammarsten, Gilbert, Fournier, Heim, Lahmann, von Noorden, Epstein, Wair Mitchel, Salkowski, Kornauth and the rest, but not one of them ever dreamed of a perfect regenerator of the cells of the human body such as this composition, Eubiogen, affords.

The analysis of my product, shows that it is practically impossible to improve upon in life-giving, cell-generating qualities. This fact should satisfy the student. Still I will describe the ingredients a little more minutely, so that all who use it may be convinced that they are doing the best that can be done, as known to the science of to-day, to improve conditions of health for themselves and for their offspring.

As a basis, then, I use for the necessary trituration, the finest radio-active milk sugar produced, flavored with *pure* vanilla extract. The high percentage of albumen contained in it is due to the use of the most highly perfected hygienic product of albumen known to chemistry. It is chemically pure and manufactured from eggs, milk and vegetables and, therefore, absolutely free from microscopical germs, harmful to the human system.

The organic iron contained in it is obtained from the red-coloring matter of healthy ox blood, called haemin, examined and tested. For the nerve material, pure lecithin or nerve fat is used, obtained from the yolks of fresh eggs.

These two products are enormously expensive. All the organic minerals are in the form of glycerophosphates, and the milk sugar necessary for making a perfect trituration is radio-active, as explained before.

To make the whole product as digestible and assimilable as possible, I use the best material known, that is, Taka and Malt diastase.

It is made palatable through the use of genuine van Houten's cocoa in chocolate form. It will remain in good condition an unlimited length of time when kept in a dry, cool place. No drugs of any kind are used. This I guarantee in the fullest sense of the word. The manufacturer is a renowned chemist of the highest type, and all the products are of the highest quality obtainable. This is capable of verification by any really capable authority on the chemistry of food.

In order to bring this product within the reach of all classes, the same has been compounded in three different forms:

Form aaa. contains radio-activity, haemin, lecithin, glycerophosphates and all other constituents of the highest purity.

Form aa. contains haemin, lecithin, glycerophosphates and all other constituents of the highest purity.

Form a. contains haemoglobin, glycerophosphates and all other constituents (chemically pure.)

For the use of babies and very feeble invalids, special composition B (see appendix) may take the place of Eubiogen, since it contains nearly all of its constituent elements in a form that can be assimilated by either. It will regenerate the invalid as fast as his condition will allow, and is the salvation of weak children.

(c). As to when Eubiogen should be administered, the rule is simple.

Whenever any of the Dech-Manna Compositions are given, Eubiogen should be given in smaller or larger doses, as the case may require, remembering that its most important task is to rebuild and regenerate the body so that it may readily perform its fullest functions and transmit the power unimpared to posterity.

(d). *Dose*: The dose may vary considerably, from 1 to 3 times a day. Generally a dose consists of 1 gram or one-fourth of a heaping teaspoonful.

The composition may be combined with any kind of food, or may be given in separate form with chocolate in equal parts.

There are endless ways in which my remedies may be administered, since they are merely concentrated cell-food.

It must be definitely understood at the outset that these remedies must be absolutely and entirely dissociated with the idea of so-called "medicine," prescribed by the old-school doctor, which has nothing whatsoever in common with my "remedies," since these contain the real constituents of our body-cells and *not* poisonous chemical concoctions, known as medicines, which *may* in some cases suppress symptoms, *but never will and never can remove the constitutional cause or condition of disease.*

COMPARATIVE ANALYSIS.

The Human Body consists of:

83.0%	Water	\
0.9%	Minerals	|
3.8%	Albumen	| Solid consti-tuents
2.5%	Fat	| only 17%
9.8%	Carbohydrates	|
— — —		|
100.0%		/

Eubiogen consists of:

9.0%	Minerals. (Chiefly Glycerophos-phates, Haemin or Blood-Iron and organized minerals)	10 times concentrated.
33.5%	Albumen. (Egg, Milk and Vegetable-Albumen)	9 " "
15.0%	Fats. (Chiefly Cacao, Glycerin fats, Lecithin) (Note. — Lecithin is made from fresh yolks of egg.)	6 " "
42.5%	Carbohydrates (Chiefly Malt Extract, Milk, Sugar etc.)	5 " "
— — —		Of the original amount
100.0%	Solid Constituents.	in the human body.

Note.

1 Pound of Powdered Egg-Albumen represents the total egg-albumen contents of 116 Eggs. 1 Pound of Powdered Milk-Albumen represents the total milk-albumen of 25 pints of Milk. 1 Pound of Blood-Iron represents 250 pounds of Haemoglobin.
(The cost of Haemoglobin is $4.50 per pound, the value, therefore, of 1 pound of Haemin or Blood-Iron is $1,125 —)

APPENDIX I

LIFE PRESERVERS AND ELIXIRS.

In addition to the twelve Dech-Manna Compositions mentioned before, I have composed three others that are most important and are to be used practically and in various doses; the first and the third should be used in nearly every treatment of patients suffering from constitutional diseases, while the second is the remedy which takes the place of Eubiogen when the patients are babies or very weak.

SPECIAL DECH-MANNA COMPOSITION. (A) OXYGENATOR.

This consists of radium emanation tablets or powders and the necessary bath salts for the decarbonization of the system in all cases of what is called auto-intoxication. They have a wonderful effect on the metabolism of the human organism, and increase the oxidation of all diseased cells that poison the system. The radium tablets are officially guaranteed and the bath salts are the result of many years study in balneotherapy and hydrotherapy, and have demonstrated their effectiveness by the wonderful results that have been obtained during the last thirty years. Rheumatism, gout, arterio-sclerosis, etc., cannot exist in the system when these baths have been taken for a certain length of time. I rarely undertake a treatment for disease of this kind without them.

HOW TO APPLY OXYGENATOR.

For a half or partial bath fill the bath two-thirds full of water at 90° to 98°. Use one pound of bath salts. Mix and dissolve them completely in the water. As soon as dissolved, put two of the oxygenator radium tablets into the water, one at the head and one at the foot of the bath, allowing one-half to one minute for dissolving. Mix very slowly and quietly in order not to release too much of the radium emanation.

Lie in the bath very quietly for 20 to 25 minutes, with cold compresses on the head. Then open the cold water faucet, begin to move about in the bath, sit up and wash face and chest with cold water. Let the cold water run into the bath until you notice some signs of "goose-flesh," then get out and rub down well with a good Turkish towel.

Never remain alone while taking this kind of a bath. Stop the bath immediately if any feeling of faintness is experienced. Drink a glass of Tonogen, or other refreshment.

SPECIAL DECH-MANNA COMPOSITION. (B)
EUBIOGEN LIQUID.

This composition is in liquid form and intended for babies and very feeble invalids. It contains nearly all the constituents of No. XII, Eubiogen, but in such a form that even the infant can safely partake of it, with rapid regenerative results. Thus the degeneration of inherited or predisposed conditions or weak tissues will be prevented.

Dose: From one-half to three teaspoonfuls a day, pure or diluted in milk, according to the individual directions given. As a fermentative agent I know of nothing better, and through the formation of gases, acidity of the stomach will be prevented, perfect digestion assured and consequently health and normal conditions restored.

SPECIAL DECH-MANNA COMPOSITION. (C)
TONOGEN.

As a beverage Tonogen scientifically speaking, stands at the head of all chemical achievements in drinks. Therapeutically, there is nothing that could be more beneficial to the human system. It contains the fundamental constituents of normal blood and nerve cells in such form that even the weakest and most sensitive digestion will readily respond to its influence. This compound is absolutely free from all deleterious chemicals; as a tonic it is stimulating and strengthening and as a beverage it is so palatable that few will hesitate to pronounce its taste delicious.

In all cases of acute febrile diseases, also in chronic forms of these diseases, as well as in climatic fevers, it is wonderfully effective in supporting the healing process of nature.

From a physiologico-chemical standpoint, it has been thus described:

Tonogen is the acme of chemical perfection, both as a tonic and as a beverage. It is the captured and crystalized outcome of years of scientific observation focussed upon the true ingredients of healthy blood cells as viewed from both the theoretical and practical biological standpoint. It represents, in fact, a life study of the science of life, in a concrete form of body-cell invigorator suitable to all mankind, from earliest infancy to advancing age, and this of a nature equally digestible and assimilable to both. After but a brief experience of this seductive beverage, it may speedily be felt how, once digested and assimilated, it courses through the lymph channels and lacteal vessels and, by the familiar route of the Chyle passes into the heart, where joined with the blood of that organ, it produces a sensation of liquifaction. In its course, by way of the arteries, it gradually reaches the external glands, warms the limbs and, in a manner electrifies them. In the body, it suffuses the pancreas and other glands and the intestines, mingles with the fluids existing in the glands and with the oily salts of the bile; and whatever impurities (autotoxins), may be there it drives in the form of excrement and urine completely out of the body. Thus in its free and ample scope is all the ground of all the intricate vital processes of physiology covered in its course and the active principles of the excretions of skin, kidneys and intestines are made visible at a glance.

In combination with Plasmogen, taken alternately, it is really indespensable in all the diseases mentioned above. Many a life has been saved through the use of this combination. It is one of my standard home remedies, and my own family would not think of allowing themselves to be without it for a single day, for, as they say, one never knows when it may be required.

Dose: One teaspoonful tonogen with three teaspoonfuls of granulated sugar in a tumbler of water, to be taken slowly, once or twice daily. In cases of diabetes and arterio-sclerosis the dose should be 20 to 25 drops tonogen in a teaspoonful of milk sugar 1 to 3 times daily. Pregnancy is a contra-indication to the use of tonogen.

APPENDIX II.

The following compositions are also used especially in specific cases.

(D). Tea. Diabetic. *Dechmann.*

Description: Compound of many herbs (powdered) found beneficial to the diabetic system.

(E). Tea. Laxagen. *Kneipp.*

Description: Compound of several herbs (powdered) approved by the celebrated Kneipp in cases of chronic constipation.

(F). Salve. Lenicet. *Reiss.*

Description: The most beneficial salve in case of inflamed wounds, boils or exanthematous eruptions.

(G). Massage Emulsion. *Dechmann.*

Description: Consists of the finest ethereal oils and other ingredients useful and valuable, yet absolutely harmless, in case of nerve or muscular pains, applied as a liniment.

(H). Propionic acid.

Description: The product of various herbs known for their high percentage of propionic acid; applied in case of catarrh in the form of atomized steam.

(I). Oxygen Powder. *Hensel.*

Description: A composition of sugar, gum tragacanth (traganth) and citric acid, used in the form of lemonade in case of high carbonic acid poisoning.

(J). Anti-Phosphate. *Dechmann.*

(Otherwise termed "Negative Compound.")

Description: Contains all basic salts as sulphates, thus acting as the governor of a machine; that is it prevents the accumulation of too much phosphate in the blood, which would promote the formation of all fungus growths. (See paragraph in the article, "Importance of the Mineral Constituents in our food").

A copy of my wholesale price list as given in 1915—before we entered the war—may give you a fair idea of the price of my compositions. Since that time, most of the ingredients of these remedies have increased from four to ten times in value. The reader can easily judge therefrom of the fairness of the present values. I may say that most of the compositions are listed at only one-fourth to one-third advance, notwithstanding the high cost of chemicals. This fact will absolve me, I think, of any tendency to profiteering.

PRICE-LIST DECH-MANNA COMPOSITIONS.

No.		Per oz.	Per lb.
I.	Plasmogen	$0.75	$ 8.00
II.	Lymphogen	1.00	10.67
III.	Neurogen	1.50	16.00
IV.	Osseogen	1.00	10.67
V.	Muscogen	1.00	10.67
VI.	Mucogen	1.00	10.67
VII.	Dento & Ophthogen	1.50	16.00
VIII.	Capillogen	1.50	16.00
IX.	Dermogen	1.50	16.00
X.	Gelatinogen	1.50	16.00
XI.	Cartilogen	1.50	16.00
XII.	Eubiogen	2.00	21.35
	Same with sacch. lact. radio	2.50	26.67

A reduction of 33⅓% on the prices per pound
will be allowed on all the above products as
quoted in the second column.

A.	Radio emanation tablet (5,000 volts);				
	Per tablet				$ 1.50
	Bath salts, original composition, lb.				1.00
B.	Eubiogen Liquid	(a)	oz. 0.75	(b)	oz. 1.00
			pt. 8.00		pt. 10.67
C.	Tonogen	(a)	oz. 0.50	(b)	oz. 0.75

			pt. 5.33		pt. 8.00
J.	Anti-Phosphate	(a)	oz. 0.50	(b)	oz. 0.75
			lb. 5.33		lb. 8.00

Copies of the Handbook "Dare To Be Healthy"
Second Edition, may be procured at 75c for the
paper-bound edition and $1.50 for the
leather-bound edition.

PHYSICAL TREATMENT.

As I have already stated, it is necessary in disease to assist the process of regulating the circulation and opening the body to the full benefit of the dietetic and nutritive salts treatment by applying a number of physical treatments, in each case, which, for convenience sake, I have divided into ten different groups, some of which may need to be applied simultaneously in certain cases.

They are as follows:

23. Ablutions with vinegar and water,   1 part vinegar, 2 parts water.

24. Abdominal packs, vinegar and water,   dito

25. Partial packs:
(a) Vinegar and water,   dito
(b) Radium and salts.

26. Partial packs:
(a) Arms.
(b) Legs.
(c) Neck.
(d) Shoulder.

27. Three-quarter packs, vinegar and water,   dito

28. Gymnastics.

29. Massage.

30. Breathing Exercises.

31. Oxygenator Baths.

32. Radium and Salt Baths.
(a) Half.

(b) Whole.

NOTE — **The Vinegar** indicated to be used for these treatments, and in all similar treatments, packs, or ablutions, prescribed, is the natural, or what is known as "Apple Cider Vinegar." The manufactured or ordinary table vinegar, as made from chemicals, is not suitable for the purpose.

From these groups a treatment is usually prescribed in each and every case of disease.

The importance of ablutions especially packs is so great that it is necessary to give further explanations concerning them:

In a general way, it is necessary to apply a bath or an ablution (See Form 23) when the test with the thermometer, usually applied under the tongue, in arm-pit or in the rectum, shows that the temperature of the patient exceeds 100 degrees. The patient grows restless, his skin feels dry and the pulse, which regularly is 70 to 80 with adults, 90 to 100 with children, and about 130 with infants, shows an increased speed. As soon as these symptoms appear, they indicate that the immediate cooling off of the body by means of a bath, an ablution or a pack is necessary. Adults will always show the desire for such instinctively.

In extreme cases baths or ablutions should be administered several times every day.

Healthy people perspire as soon as they become too hot. This means that they cool off through the evaporation of the perspiration. This is supplemented by the bath and its cooling effect; balancing the higher temperature of the body with the lower temperature of the water, brings this about. The blood which flows towards the skin during the bath is cooled off, and returns in this condition to the interior of the body, and is immediately followed by other quantities of blood.

Since the blood circulates through the body about twice every minute, the cooling takes place from 20 to 24 times during a bath, lasting from 10 to 12 minutes. This explains the soothing and cooling effect of the bath on the waves of blood and the nerves, which are irritated by the increased temperature.

At the same time the bath opens the pores which assist in the excretion of degenerated matter produced by the disease, and fosters the reception of oxygen.

It is a natural function of the body that an increased flow of the warming blood flies always to any region of the body which is assailed by external cold, so that such parts may not become too cold or, in common parlance, may not "catch" cold.

This explains why the hands get red and hot after throwing snow-balls, the feet burn after a cold foot bath.

As soon as the body, which is hot with fever, is put into the cool bath, the first effect is that the blood-vessels of the skin contract under the cooling influence. The blood recedes. Soon, however, it streams with renewed energy to the skin to defeat the cold. The first action,—the recession of the blood,—is followed by reaction or increased activity of circulation towards the skin. This removes the pressure of the blood upon the overburdened internal organs, such as the brain, the lungs and the heart. The blood is diverted.

For ablutions the water should be cool or lukewarm, the exact temperature to be determined by the strength of the patient. Some vinegar should be added to the water, taking two parts water and one part vinegar.

To accustom children to the use of water and ablutions is one of the important duties of motherhood.

A healthy child should be washed once every day with water at 59 degrees to 64 degrees. The best way to wash the child is to put two chairs in front of its bed. On one of them place the vessel with the necessary water, on the other place the child, after it has been disrobed in bed, in a standing position, so that it can be supported with the back of the chair. The ablution is performed by means of strong application with the hands, dipped into the water, and is repeated several times. Then the shirt is put on again, and the child is allowed to stay well covered in bed for another 15 minutes.

Children must become accustomed to gargling as early as possible, and to draw water up through the nose, or to remove it from the mouth through the nose. This is very valuable and facilitates the treatment of children in case of disease.

VINEGAR PACKS.

It appears opportune at this juncture, and before entering upon the detailed description of the modern healing system of Vinegar Packs, included in the prescribed course of Physical Treatments which follow, to make a few rational remarks illustrative of the physical significance and scientific basis of a branch of therapy which largely amongst the laity, through ignorance, and more so amongst the regular medical fraternity, for reasons of their own, is too frequently lightly regarded by the one and diplomatically depreciated by the other.

In this manner one of the most potent and logical modern factors in the healing of disease would be conveniently consigned to the back ground in company with other simple *but unremunerative* truths, but for the timely intervention of the new and enlightened school of independent medicine of which the Biological or Hygienic Dietetic Method of Healing is the outcome.

The wonderful efficacy of natural Vinegar upon the organism and its employment in the form of Vinegar Packs and compresses dates back probably to the early traditions of the healing art, but scientific analysis of its subtle operation upon the system through the vital fluid has been left for the scientific research of today to determine.

To those of the public — or the profession — therefore, who are not conversant with the subject the following notes may be valuable as descriptive of the why and wherefore of the use of Vinegar.

It will be admitted, I think, that one of the most prolific sources of disease, in innumerable forms, is that of congestion of blood. The greatest danger of such congestion is inflammation. Should inflammation occur in or near a vital organ and fail to be promptly reduced and its cause (coagulation) removed, the result is decomposition — and decomposition, if not arrested means death.

The most valuable — I might almost say infallible — remedy known, even to the greatest accepted authorities of physiology, for the prevention of inflammation is acetic acid in diluted form, or, in a word, Vinegar, as a restorer of the fluidity of the blood.

Inflammation is the result of coagulation of the blood-albumen; congestion is its sequal, inflammation and decomposition of the tissues its climax. The last is nearly always fatal.

The manifest object therefore to be achieved in all such cases is to restore the normal fluidity and circulation of the blood without unduly taxing any vital organ. Thus, for instance, hot packs on the feet draw the blood towards the feet, where no vital organs exist. Hot packs act as an absorbent, by suction; cold packs, on the affected place, act in inverse ratio as an expelling force. The two operating conjointly promote full circulation and extend the absorbing tendency to the whole system.

Ice, on the other hand, though not infrequently prescribed, is too strong a force. It contracts the blood vessels, arrests normal circulation, and in many cases is the direct cause of death. This is attested by the teaching of physiological law which maintains that any part of the human system which is not fed by fresh oxygenous blood *must decompose*.

Packs, of course, must be regulated in accordance with the vital strength of the patient, as indicated by the physician; for in the course of the excretion of morbid matter through the pores, under the influence of the packs, a certain proportion of accompanying healthy substance is necessarily exuded simultaneously, with a slightly weakening tendency. This however can be promptly and effectively replaced by proper alimentation, or food selection in accordance with the Dech-Manna Diet System already particularized.

One other matter it is advisable to deal with in advance and that is the *Nature of the Vinegar to be employed for Packs*.

It must be borne in mind that for this purpose an absolutely pure natural product should be obtained.

I recommend, in the first place a genuine *Apple Cider Vinegar*; for apples not alone contain the pure acetic acid but also some five or six other fruit acids which are so beneficial for the purpose of keeping the blood at normal temperature and normal fluidity, and contain also a considerable amount of the essentials known under the head of vitamines.

As a secondary alternative I would recommend *Wine Vinegar* for the same purpose.

The manufacturers vinegar product—*Acetic acid, should never the used* as it contains, very frequently, harmful ingredients.

It should never be forgotten that the substances used for the purpose of packs, and thus absorbed into the system, become a part of the blood and therefore cannot be too pure.

The reader will doubtless observe from the foregoing demonstration that the Dechmann System of Therapy differs materially from the science of the Old-School of Medicine in that it is not based upon evanescent theories of hairsplitting philosophy but upon the solid basis of cold-blooded fact.

Why then, the reader will inquire, should so wonderful and at the same time *simple, inexpensive and easily applied remedy* be treated by "the faculty" with an affectation of indulgent toleration, ridicule or "damning with faint praise."

To this riddle there are two solutions—neither of them very creditable to those concerned.

On the one hand, only crass ignorance of some of the most important facts of physiology and physiological chemistry could account for it. And, it must be borne in mind that in the course of the prolific verbosity of pontificated dogma which has graced the scroll of medical science, whole libraries have been written—and ably written, too—by skillful pens for the sole purpose of covering the simple nudity of the agnostic position of science—the dreaded, confidence-shattering admission: "I don't know."

Failing this solution there is, unfortunately, but one alternative and that a singularly distasteful one to entertain; namely, to attribute the unpopularity of this splendid gift of Nature to unprofessional considerations on the part of an apothecary-loving profession.

The employment of vinegar is, as I have said, a royal remedy, ready to the hand of any man and at little or no expense, and it needs no "learned" interpretation.

It is consequently beyond the omnivorous talons of "the trade."

Would it be unkind to say: "Hinc illae lachrymae"?

THE PACKS.

The packs mentioned as physical treatment, under Nos. 24, 25, 26 and 27, are of the greatest importance, and in fact I never undertake the treatment of any disease whatsoever without applying them as the most effective means of restoring proper circulation of the blood and removing diseased matter from the body, which is the only way to bring about a real and definite cure.

The effect of the pack is the cooling of the blood.

The temperature of the pack is 50 degrees and more below the temperature of the blood.

In the first place this brings about quiet after unrest.

Through the action of the body, which sends a large quantity of blood to the places which are touched by the cool compresses, a certain surplus of heat is created which is transferred to the compresses and retained by them as moist warmth.

Under this influence the blood-vessels of the skin extend and absorb blood more freely, which is thus diverted from the important internal organs to the skin. In all cases of fever the diseased matter is dissolved in the hot feverish blood and circulates in and with it. The evaporation of the skin is increased, and with it the diseased matter is absorbed by the compresses, which consequently diffuse an unpleasant odor when removed, and when cleansed, give to the water a muddy appearance. Thus it may be observed to what extent the pack removes diseased matter from the body.

Packs must be changed as soon as they cease to give comfort to the patient, and make him too warm. Highly flushed cheeks, increasing temperature and unrest are sure signs that the pack requires to be changed, and in case of high fever this may happen after 20 to 30 minutes.

For short packs, such as are prescribed in all inflammatory and feverish diseases, water at from 59 degrees to 64 degrees is used.

A piece of linen cloth is folded from 4 to 8 times, wrung out, but not too much, and then covered with moderately thick folds of woollen cloth. The stronger the patient and the higher the fever, the thicker should be the pack.

For infants a double linen strip is sufficient.

The faster the fever and inflammation recede, the longer may the pack last, up to three hours. The convalescent will enjoy the moist warmth, under the influence of which still existing diseased material is thoroughly dissolved and completely excreted. The dissolving effect of packs of long duration is most noticeable in chronic diseases.

Through the penetrating effect of the moist warmth on the body or parts thereof, deposited diseased matter is dissolved, and dislodged, existing excoriations are disintegrated, and withdrawn into the circulating blood, and thus excreted.

The dissolving packs of long duration must be applied somewhat thinner than the cooling ones (from 1 to 3 folds); they must be wrung out more vigorously, and covered more closely.

If a pack should be applied for the sake of prevention of disease, it may be put on in the evening and remain all night. In the beginning of fever, while it remains moderate, the patient can endure the pack for from 2 to 2½ hours.

Biological hygienic therapy rejects the external application of ice, for it causes severe congestion of the blood. Extensive application of the ice pouch causes more or less paralysis of the nerves, which in many cases prevents recovery and even causes chronic disease or fatal results. The biological hygienic treatment desires *to moderate inflammation only*, to the degree that it should lose its dangerous character, but it leaves to the body its power *to remove, through the process of inflammation, alien and diseased matter, and to absorb and gradually carry away the products of inflammation through the blood current.*

Paralysis of the vocal cords, of the muscles of the eye, of the nerves of hearing, the exudations from the nose and eyes after diphteria, meningitis and scarlet fever, adhesions, suppurations after pneumonia and other forms of inflammatory disease, are often the *consequences of the use of ice*, because the products of inflammation are not absorbed, and the ice paralyzes the neighbouring nerves.

Inflammations, which are suppressed by medicine or ice, must renew themselves; since the causes, the alien matter (auto toxins), as well as the products of inflammation remain in the body and are not thoroughly excreted.

To apply water, on the contrary, quickly removes not only the inflammation, but its causes and eventual consequences. The organs which have been inflamed do not show any further inclination to renewed inflammation.

In no case will a chronic ailment be the consequence of an acute disease, provided the same is dealt with in a natural way, according to the principles of biological hygienic treatment.

In order to bring about the complete excretion of all autotoxins and, in case of inflammation, the complete absorption of all products thereof, it is necessary to continue the lengthy packs even during the period of convalescence, and not to stop immediately the fever and inflammation have somewhat disappeared. This is a mistake which is frequently committed, and the fault is then laid at the door of the biological hygienic system. Any relapse, or succeeding illness, will be avoided by continuing the packs for four to six weeks after the disease has been cured, applying them during the night and at first also during the day-time, from two to three hours.

While most people understand the cooling effect of a pack, *the important diverting, dissolving and excreting effect is rarely understood.* Few people understand why ablutions, abdominal and leg packs are prescribed in case of inflammation of the eyes; why, in case of ulcers, besides compresses on the part affected, nightly abdominal packs and ablutions in the morning, are considered indispensable; and why, in case of inflammation of *one* leg, the healthy leg is also subjected to a pack.

And yet the explanation is very simple, rational and logical.

In limiting packs, in case of inflammation, to the inflamed part only, the blood current would be directed mainly to the one place, and the excretion of autotoxins from the body would only occur in the inflamed place. The blood would carry all diseased matter principally to the diseased spot and deposit it there. The inflamed organ would thus be burdened with work which it simply would not be able to perform. The effect is far otherwise when the pressure of blood into the diseased part is moderated, if the dissolution and excretion of the matter that causes the disease, takes place, not in one spot only, but is distributed over the entire body. If the entire skin comes into action, the entire body participates in the healing process. In biological hygienic-dietetic practice it is, consequently, not sufficient to treat the one diseased organ only. In all diseases *the co-operation of the entire body in a general treatment, remains the main issue of the biological, hygienic therapy*. It regards the human body, as so often stated, purely as a unit, and knows neither specialist nor special cures. This is the key to its success.

IMPORTANT GENERAL ADVICE.

For use in packs take coarse, previously used and loosely woven linen, which readily absorbs water and clings closely to the body.

After each pack the linen must be rinsed well and boiled and the woollen material or blanket must be thoroughly aired. From time to time the woollen covering must be washed, or chemically cleaned, if possible.

Raw silk is an excellent substitute for linen. It clings well to the body, does not cause any discomfort, and has an excellent absorbing quality for water and other substances.

The proper application of the pack is of course of great importance. Adults can easily apply many of the packs without assistance, but generally speaking a third person is necessary, whether in the case of children or patients. It is consequently advisable for every mother to become thoroughly familiar with the methods of applying packs, and she should always have the necessary material on hand. It should be cut to the proper size, and there should be duplicates of each piece for the necessary changes. The approximate measurements for adults are:

	Width	Length
Neck pack	5"	40" to 60"
Shoulder pack	10"	40"
Abdominal pack	28"	40" to 60"
Breast or stomach pack	16"	52" to 60"
"T" pack	16"	52" to 60"
Cross piece alone	5"	24"
The shawl	32" to 40"	32" to 40"
Scotch pack (undivided)	16"	80" to 100"
Same for children	10" to 16"	60" to 80"
Calf pack	24"	26"

Leg pack	24"	30"
Three-quarter pack	56"	52" to 60"
Whole pack	68"	80"

The measurements for children are accordingly shorter and narrower.

As to the application of packs, a mother can learn a great deal by experimenting on her own body. Packs at night are by no means detrimental to adults, and the application of a regular abdominal pack, a three-quarter pack, and a whole pack once a week or once every two weeks is decidedly advantageous. Three-quarter and whole packs should be occasionally tried on the body of children with dry linen so that in case of disease the mother will be a well trained nurse, at least in this respect.

To go about the application of the pack quietly and without much talking is very comforting to the patient, who usually grows excited during the procedure.

In case of acute feverish disease the packs and the changes must be applied very quickly, so that the patient will not catch cold. While, as a rule, the patient should not be disturbed in a quiet sleep, unconsciousness or delirium must not prevent change of the pack.

Packs should be applied so as not to cause any creases which may hurt the patient.

The temperature of the water used for packs should be as follows:

For the cooling packs, 59 degrees to 64 degrees.

For dissolving packs, 64 degrees to 71 degrees.

The higher temperature is used in the treatment of infants, nervous and anaemic persons.

In chronic diseases a gradual return to a lower temperature by about 2½ degrees per week is advisable.

No packs or compresses should be put on when parts of the body are cold. In such cases the parts in question must first be warmed.

The linen should be wrung out less for short cooling compresses than for dissolving packs of longer duration.

Cooling compresses must be changed as soon as the patient indicates that he feels oppressed or irritated by the heat.

As a general rule, packs on the legs may be left on feverish patients twice as long as packs on the upper parts of the body.

No fever being apparent, the abdominal pack may be changed after about 2½ hours, the leg pack after 5 hours, and even not at all during the night. Packs should be renewed according to requirements of the individual patient, not in accordance with fixed rules.

Great care must be exercised to fasten the packs well and tightly. This is usually done with good strong safety pins; these should be fastened perpendicularly, or at right angles to the length of the material.

When changing the pack on feverish patients who are to receive an ablution or a bath two or three times a day, all pins must be loosened under the bedcovers so that the pack may be removed quickly.

If ablutions only are to be given, the pack is removed gradually as the respective parts of the body are to be washed.

When the fever is moderate, there should be ablutions morning and evening, or a bath in the morning and an ablution in the evening.

When packs are applied only at night, patients require only an ablution in the morning.

If the packs are not renewed, an ablution must follow the removal. This refreshes and strengthens the skin, closes the wide open pores and prevents taking cold.

Dissolving packs, if annoying at night, may be removed under the bedcovers without an ablution.

If the pack is changed without intervening ablution, the new pack must be ready to be applied before the old, hot one, is taken off.

While in a pack, the patient should not leave his bed, not even for the purpose of urinating or for stool.

GENERAL RULES.

The following general rules must be applied in connection with the directions given anon for packs during different diseases.

In case of inflammation, the inflamed spot is cooled off by local compresses, and diverting packs of longer duration are applied on other parts of the body.

For instance, in case of inflammation of the brain or tonsils.

The first step is to cool off the blood which flows to the neck and head by short-time compresses on the neck and on the cervix. At the same time an attempt must be made to divert it through lengthier packs on the abdomen, the legs and the wrists, thereby to prevent a further delivery of diseased matter to the centre of inflammation. The solution and excretion of diseased matter from other points than the inflamed spots will thereby be effected, and these will be unburdened and calmed accordingly.

In case of inflammation of the organs of the breast (lungs, heart), the blood is diverted to the abdomen, legs and lower arms through long-time packs, and the upper parts of the breast are cooled with short compresses.

If the inflammation has its seat in the abdomen, this must be cooled off, while the diversion with longer-time packs is made to the legs and arms.

Ulcers are treated by applying extremely hot compresses, which are frequently changed, and the surrounding parts are cooled off and diversion is effected through nightly packs on the abdomen and on the legs. The hot compresses dissolve the diseased matter, so that the ulcer opens. Thereupon cool compresses of 71 degrees to 64 degrees are applied and allowed to remain for 2½ to 3 hours, which will effect quick healing without the necessity of an operation.

The main rule is never to divert towards a vital organ of the body, such as the lungs or heart; thus, in case of inflammation of the head, diversion must be attempted, not to the breast, but to the arms and legs.

ABDOMINAL PACK (24)

The abdominal pack should be applied on infants and children whenever they show signs of illness in any way, and naturally, in cases of summer complaints, measles, scarlet fever, diphtheria, whooping cough, pneumonia, typhoid fever, in which cases a pack should be applied during the entire course of the illness with slight intermissions only.

As in acute diseases, it is also applied in chronic ones. (See descriptions to follow). Its early application will often serve to prevent serious sickness.

The abdominal pack reaches from the level of the base of the breast bone to the hips. It is made from a piece of linen crash about 12 inches in width which must cover the space from 6 inches below the arm-pits to the hips, while its length must be such that it can encircle the body, overlap upon the abdomen and be secured with tapes at the left side. A further piece of soft linen is needed to pass between the legs, to be fastened to the former, back and front, with safety-pins. The next requirement is a piece of woollen cloth, or blanket, folded double or treble as required, in breadth, about 6 inches wider than the linen crash and of equal length, with a shorter woollen strip for between the thighs, attached like the linen, back and front. For children a linen towel etc. with the accompanying woollen coverings, will be found, as a rule, sufficient; for infants, a properly folded piece of old linen. The linen as well as the woollen material must be properly folded before the pack is made, and measured, so that the patient need not be kept waiting while the pack is being placed on the body.

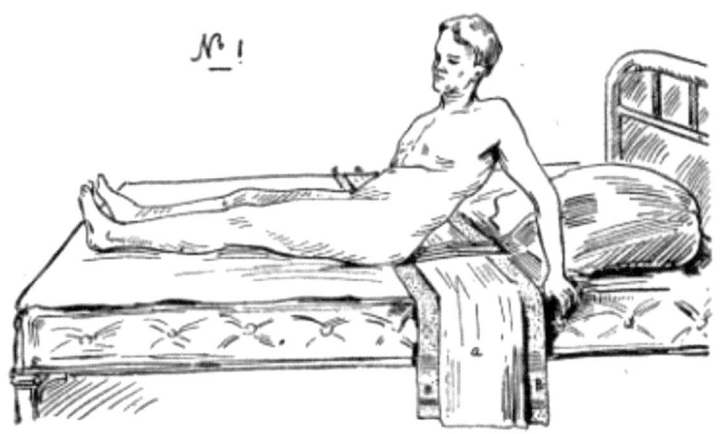

The above cut shows how to apply the abdominal pack on an adult patient.

The linen is saturated in two parts of water with one part of vinegar, at 64 to 75 degrees Fahrenheit, well wrung out, and is placed on the woollen material in such a way that the latter extend about 2 to 3 inches on the upper and lower edge. The pack is now placed around the back of the patient, who sits in bed or is held in position by another. The patient's shirt is lifted and he is laid down on the moist linen, which is then quickly raised on both sides and folded over the abdomen. The same is done with the woollen material, which is then fastened tightly in the middle, the upper and lower corners with three safety pins. Then the shirt is pulled down and the patient is warmly covered.

In individual cases it is advisable sometimes to divide the pack into a back and front compress of greater proportions.

In such cases the woollen cloth, which is used for the abdominal pack is placed underneath the patient as before. A towel is folded 6 to 8 times, so that it will grow warm slowly and thus may remain on the body for a longer time. This is placed under the back of the patient. Then two properly folded towels, which are not wrung out very thoroughly, are put on the abdomen, and tucked down a little on both sides. The woollen cloth is thereupon fastened so as to keep the compresses in place, the arrangement being otherwise exactly as before. In such cases the back compress only needs to be changed every 2 to 3 hours, even in case of severe fever. The front towels may be changed several times in the meantime.

Since this system permits the application of the pack without disturbing the patient and making him sit up too often, it is very desirable in cases of severe illness.

The undivided pack is often very uncomfortable for patients suffering from respiratory complaints.

It is better to treat very excitable patients with front compresses only.

When the stomach pack only is prescribed, as in catarrhal and nervous, stomach or liver complaints, which pack may be worn during the night as well as the day, a long, wide mesh shawl, with a bandage, 7 to 8 inches in width at each end, is most servicable, as it will reach around the body 4 or 5 times. In order to exclude the air as much as possible, the moist compress is first applied, and then the shawl is placed around the body in such a way that each succeeding turn covers the previous one to about one-half, in bandage form.

THE CROSS PACK (25)

This is applied in case of men's diseases and women's diseases of the sexual organs. To the woollen material and the linen crash of the abdominal pack, another piece, about half as long and about 7 inches wide, is sewed or pinned before application, in the form of a T.

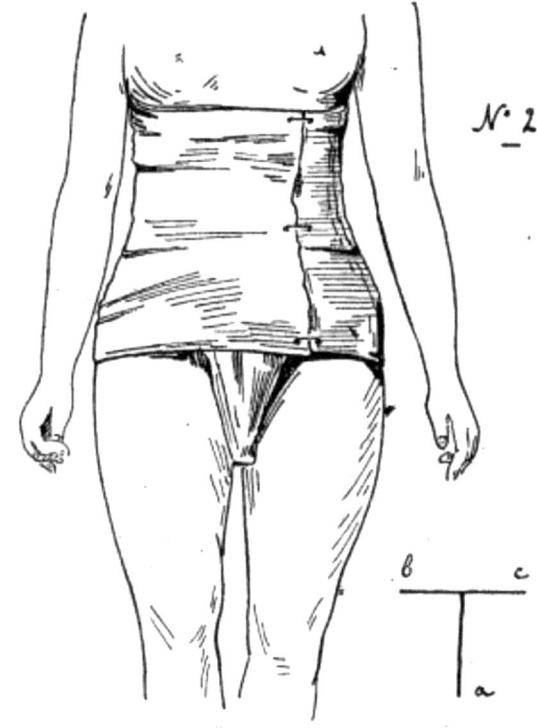

Before the two ends of the abdominal pack are folded over on the front of the abdomen, the narrower piece is drawn up between the legs from behind, so that the end of it can be fastened to the two sides of the abdominal part of the pack that are folded over in front.

As shown above, the abdominal pack must reach down as far as possible, and if a patient is unable to stand both packs, the moist part of the abdominal pack may be omitted, and only the regular pack over the sexual organs and the woollen part over the abdomen applied.

In case the cross piece is for the purpose of cooling and contracting, it must be frequently renewed.

Women should accompany the ablutions mornings and evenings with injections of lukewarm water at 71 degrees to 82 degrees, and men should make ablutions of the sexual parts 5 to 6 times a day with water at 64 degrees to 71 degrees.

The cross pack has the advantage of gradually putting back into normal position, the female organs, if they are in any way displaced.

These packs will help to cure cases of leukorrhoea and gonorrhoea, locally too, without operations or the application of poisons, especially if applied at an early stage.

LEG PACKS (26)

These are applied in a similar way to the abdominal pack.

A towel or linen is doubled, moistened, and placed upon the woollen cloth, so that the woollen material extends about two inches beyond the upper and lower edges of the towel. These are laid together under one of the patient's legs, covering it from the middle of the thigh to the ankle, turned up from both sides and fastened with three safety pins. The other leg is packed in the same way, each one separately.

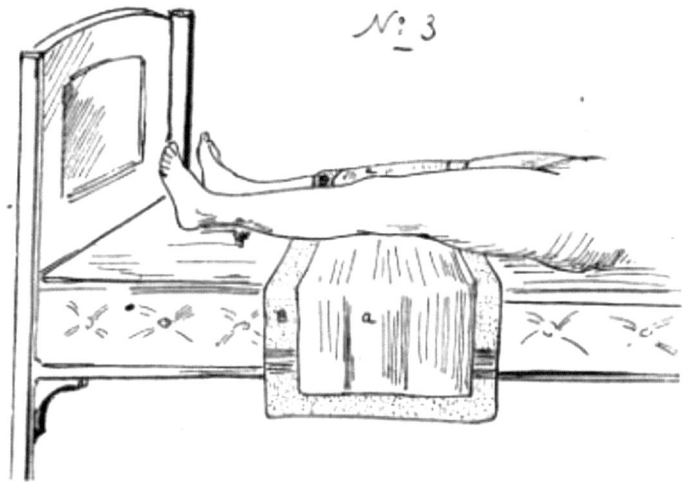

In like manner partial packs of the calves or the feet are applied. In all of these cases it is more expedient and comfortable to use "knit" packs. Cotton stockings of suitable length from which the foot has been removed, should take the place of the linen or towel in the packs previously described. They are moistened and covered with woollen stockings of corresponding length. The foot parts are to be used only for foot packs in a similar way. The woollen stocking should be as loose and comfortable as possible. In case of bent legs (through gout or otherwise) the moistened linen is wrapped around the leg like a bandage, and then a woollen bandage is wound over it.

In cases of severe fever the wrists are also packed, no woollen cover, however, being necessary in this case.

The leg pack has, in the first place, a diverting and consequently a calming effect. It is, therefore, of the highest value, next to the abdominal, cross, neck and shoulder packs, in all feverish and especially all chronic cases of disease where congestion in the head and breast, with consequent dizziness, headache, insomnia, pains in the lungs and heart, must be removed; moreover, in chronic cases, they assist in the effects of the abdominal pack.

Foot packs, that is, wet stockings, have a very favorable action upon headache, toothache and earache, and are best applied during the night. If they excite the patient too much, they may easily be taken off during the night; otherwise they should be followed by a cold ablution of the feet in the morning. Nervous patients are usually unable to stand the wet stockings, which only work well if the feet become warm quickly, which, as a rule, is not the case in feverish illnesses.

Patients who suffer from cold feet should take a steam foot bath before applying cold foot packs.

Since the legs and the feet develop less heat than the abdomen, leg and foot packs do not require as thick material as abdominal packs, and are changed less frequently. They are best applied when the fever is at its height, in the late afternoon and at night. In case leg packs are continued for a long while, the legs show decreasing inclination to grow sufficiently warm. Whenever this occurs, leg packs must be discontinued, or the packed legs must be warmed in an artificial manner.

The diverting wrist packs are of special value, especially in all acute diseases of the lungs (inflammations, bleedings, hemorrhages) and the heart.

NECK PACK (26)

This is made by folding a piece of linen fourfold, long enough to reach twice around the neck. It is dipped in the vinegar-water at from 59 degrees to 64 degrees, placed around the neck and some woollen material wound over it, covering well the moist linen.

The neck pack has its effect on the inside of the neck in case of tonsilitis, croup, etc.

If stiffness of the neck, headache or similar pains are felt after its use, the moist linen should not be extended to the back part of the neck but only the front and sides.

Where the effect is to be extended to the trachea and its branches, the bronchia and the tips of the lungs, especially in the case of cough, it is still better to apply the following:

SHOULDER PACK (26)

For this purpose a short towel is folded into a strip of about a hand's width, extending from one of the nipples across the opposite shoulder, around the neck, to the other nipple.

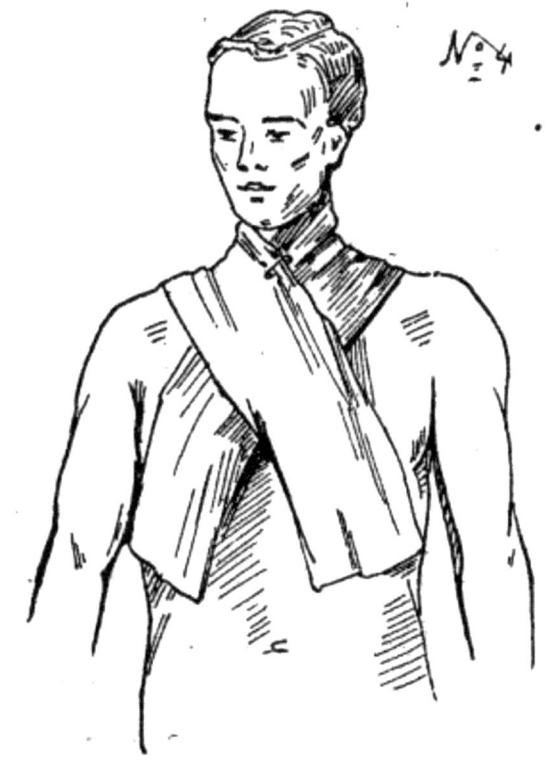

A woollen shawl or fabric, fastened together with a safety pin, must cover the moist towel completely. The shoulder pack is always applied together with the abdominal pack. It is put on first, and the two ends are pulled under the abdominal pack, and then fastened.

No 5

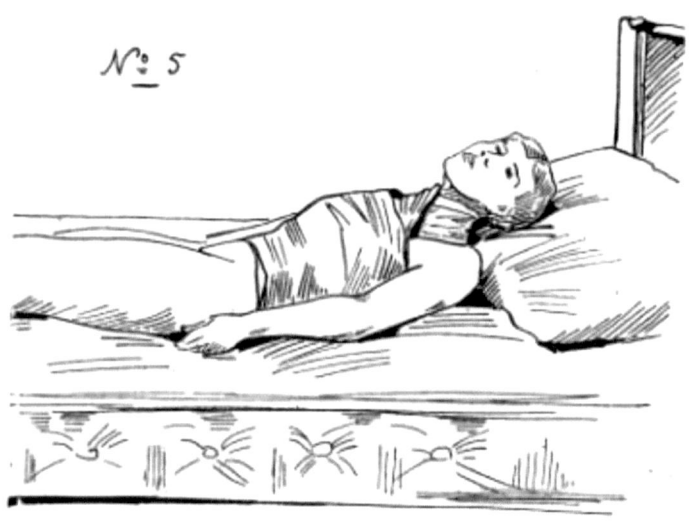

THE SCOTCH PACK (26)

The Scotch pack is of the greatest advantage in all diseases of the trachea and the lungs, also in case of whooping cough.

Two towels are sewn together lengthwise and, as a moist pack, are placed over the breast of the patient so that the seam will be in the center. The ends are crossed over the back, one end is brought forward over the left and one over the right shoulder; then the ends are crossed once more and tucked under. A woollen shawl or covering is placed over the moist towels as usual, so that it completely covers the moist pack. The ends are tucked under the pack in front. The pack is fastened with safety pins where the ends cross.

THE DIVIDED SCOTCH PACK (26)

This pack is, in some respects better than the last, since it is less liable to form creases, and the upper portion may be changed more frequently for the purposes of cooling, than the undivided pack. It is used together with the abdominal pack.

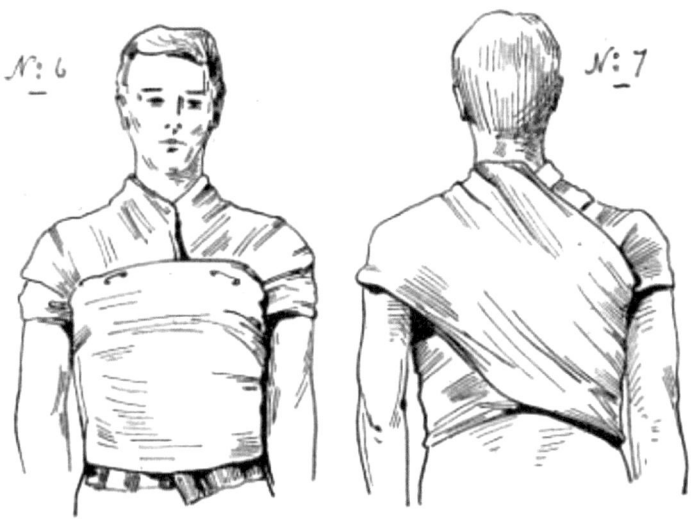

Instead of using one strip 4 to 6 inches wide, folded 4 to 6 times, as for the shoulder pack, two strips are taken. One strip is passed across each shoulder, and crossed on the breast as well as on the back. The woollen strips used for covering are of course wider and of double thickness. The ends of the two strips are drawn underneath the abdominal pack, and held by it, and the two shoulder packs may be changed as often as necessary for cooling purposes without necessitating a simultaneous change of the abdominal pack.

THE SHAWL (26)

(This is an application similar to "Kneipp's Shawl")

A large square piece of linen crash from 35 to 40 inches in width is folded into a triangle, dipped in the vinegar-water at 59 to 64 degrees, and after being wrung out, is applied diagonally round the neck. The upper part of the back, the cervix, the neck, the shoulders and the upper parts of the breast are thus covered. A woollen wrap, the ends of which are pinned together on the back, will cover the whole pack tightly.

This pack must be changed if the patient becomes too hot (after ½ to 2 hours), otherwise it may stay on all night. In case of feverish catarrh it is used together with the three-quarter pack.

Among other things the "shawl pack" causes the cooling of the blood which streams to the head. Thus its effect in case of congestion and brain trouble is explained.

Neck and shoulder packs, Scotch packs and shawl packs must always be used in connection with a diverting leg, calf or foot pack.

THE THREE-QUARTER PACK (27)

Next to the abdominal pack the three-quarter pack is one of the best applications, especially for children.

A piece of woollen cloth, or a single blanket, as long as the patient and sufficiently wide to reach all around him, is placed on the bed in such a way as to be level with the arm-pits of the patient. A bedspread of about the same size as the blanket is then dipped into cool vinegar-water, wrung out well, and placed on the blanket so that the upper edge of the latter protrudes. The patient is now laid on the bedspread so that it reaches to the arm-pits. The moist spread is then turned up on both sides, part of it is tucked between the legs, and the protruding lower end is laid on or between the feet. Thus the body, from the arms down, is completely wrapped in the wet spread, and the woollen blanket is covered over it as usual and fastened with safety pins. The patient's shirt is then adjusted. The head, the neck, the uppermost part of the breast and back are not packed. Another blanket is placed over the patient and well fastened on all sides. A pillow must be placed between the feet and the lower edge of the bed. To avoid cold feet the wet spread should reach only to the ankles, and the feet be covered with the woollen blanket, or a hot bottle placed near them.

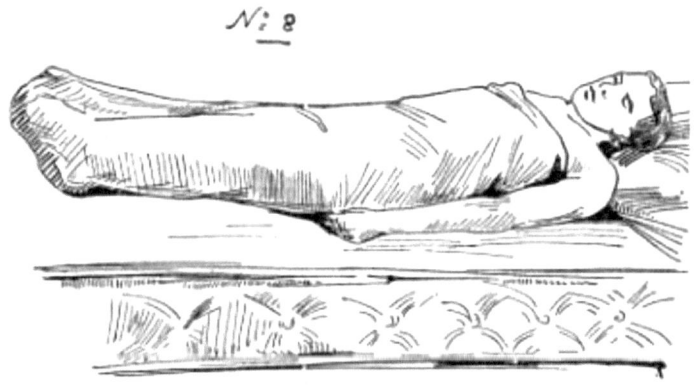

The three-quarter pack is very valuable in feverish diseases, since it takes effect on so large an area of the skin. It is also very helpful in case of meningitis and other inflammations. It should, however, not be applied by a layman, except with the greatest caution.

The inflamed parts must be covered with compresses, as in case of pneumonia and inflammation of the heart.

If three-quarter packs excite children too much, they must be replaced by abdominal and leg packs.

The patient should remain in the pack as long as he does not become too hot or restless. This may occur after 20 to 30 minutes, in case of severe fever; otherwise, the pack may last an hour or longer. The pack is very useful with children when indications of disease appear. In many cases it will develop and cure disease, such as measles, if it is properly applied for 2 to 2½ hours, and followed by a bath at 77 degrees or an ablution at 64 degrees.

When fever and inflamation begin to slacken, and also during convalescence, three-quarter or whole packs applied daily or every second day, followed by an ablution, are very useful for the purpose of solution and excretion.

In such cases the moist heat should be conserved by applying additional blankets or comforters to the limit of endurance.

THE HALF PACK (25)

The half pack is applied like the three-quarter pack, with the exception that it reaches only from the arm-pits to the knees.

It is especially necessary to close it carefully around the legs. The half pack allowing the body more freedom, it may be kept on all night.

It is most effective on the thighs in cases of sciatica. It is, however, also applied in case of febrile disease.

THE WHOLE PACK

This is applied in nearly the same way as the three-quarter pack, but includes also the arms, breast and neck.

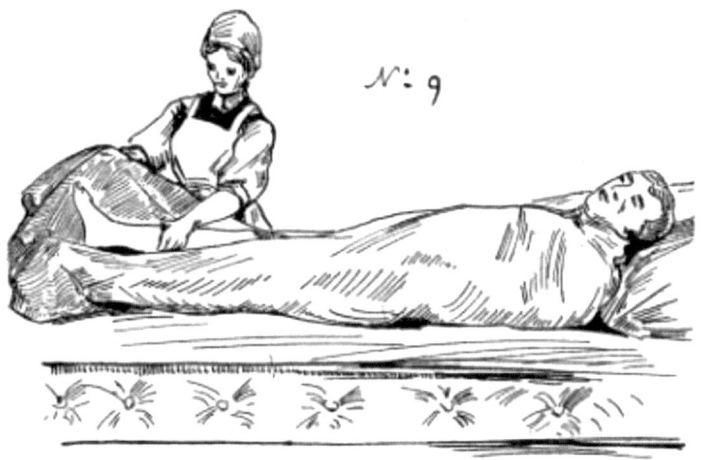

In this case the blanket must reach to above the ears. On top of the moist spread a towel is laid, which is first drawn around the abdomen. The patient's arms must be somewhat bent, so that they will not oppress the breast when packed with it. Otherwise the arms may be treated just like the legs, so that the moist spread touches them everywhere. When it is impossible to fasten the blanket at the neck with safety pins, it can be tucked firmly under both shoulders. The blanket must be drawn tightly over the shoulders and the ends tucked under the opposite shoulder. It must exceed the length of the patient by 18 inches. In case one blanket is not large enough, two must be used, one of which may be drawn down 6 inches below the other.

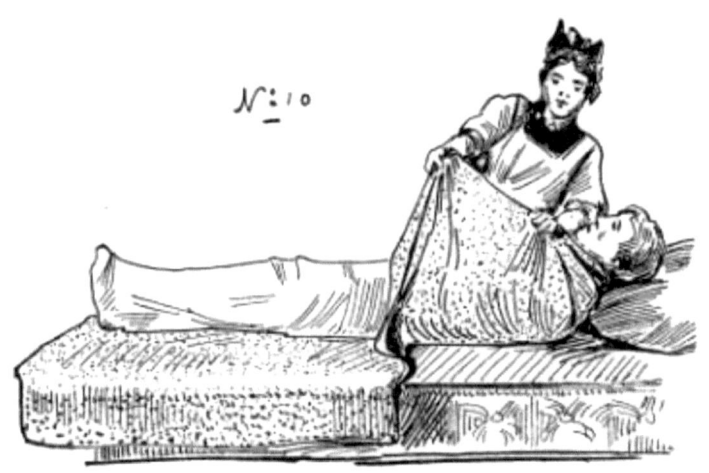

Additional blankets, pillows and comforters may be used in case of high fever.

The advice already given in regard to the differences in packs, depending on their various purposes of cooling, diverting, calming or dissolving, must also determine in this case as to the extra amount of covering. The access of cold air at the neck and legs, however, must always be carefully guarded against.

An ablution or bath must follow each whole pack.

If properly applied, the "whole pack" will be of the greatest benefit in all febrile and chronic cases.

Inflammations require partial packs, while at the same time dissolving or diverting packs of longer duration are applied to the parts of the body which are not affected.

SMALL COMPRESSES

Small compresses may be applied to any part of the body.

They reduce ulcers and slight inflammations; they dissolve coagulation in cases of rheumatism or gout, even of long standing.

A medium sized piece of linen folded six to eight times, is useful in case of toothache or earache. The compress must be covered with a woollen cloth and fastened as securely as possible. Dissolving compresses must be covered more thickly than cooling ones.

Special compresses are sometimes needed on the head, on the heart and around the neck to prevent congestions. They are covered only slightly, and like all cooling compresses, are changed as soon as they become hot.

GYMNASTICS, MASSAGE AND BREATHING EXERCISES (28, 29, 30)

The three items under "Physical Treatment": 28. *Gymnastics*, 29. *Massage* and 30. *Breathing*, require only a few explanatory remarks.

Their common object is, by means of external mechanical aid, to stimulate the circulation of the blood which is undergoing the process of regeneration. They remove obstacles to circulation and produce movements and reactions. While, in the case of massage, this external aid must, as a rule, be given by a third person in order to be effective, gymnastics and breathing exercises depend upon the patient himself. All of them, however, have the common attribute that, in order to be useful, they must be strictly individual. The old proverb: "No one thing is good for everybody," is fittingly applied in this case.

There are few things that are so much abused as this rule in regard to gymnastics. I cannot urge too strongly the importance of caution in advising such exercises. While much of what is claimed for them may be good and true, the governing question as to *what is suitable in an individual case*, can obviously not be determined by any such impersonal advice. It is the exclusive right and the duty of the attending physician to prescribe whether, and to what extent, these exercises should be applied in each case.

This is true of gymnastics even when practised by reputedly healthy people. By executing certain movements, they may develop disease and weaken certain organs, through ignorance of their abnormal condition.

In case gymnastics or breathing exercises are prescribed as part of a treatment they should be executed in strict accordance with the order of the attending hygienic-dietetic physician.

One of the great principles never to be overlooked in gymnastics is, that in order to have the desired effect they must be carried out with the greatest regularity.

As to massage, this requires knowledge of anatomy in general, and of the anatomy of the individual to be treated, in particular.

Only in this way can the desired effect be produced on certain muscles and nerves, with the further consequence that their movements promote the correct and health-giving circulation of the blood. Here again the governing factor must be the prescription of the hygienic-dietetic physician who has studied the individual case and knows the effect he wishes to produce by means of massage, and how to procure the same.

Books on massage and its general practice without knowledge of the particular case, will really accomplish nothing.

ELECTRIC VIBRATORS

In certain cases, and where it is not a question of general massage, the patient will be able to apply massage for himself according to the physician's prescription.

In this connection he will find an electric vibrator of valuable assistance. It will allow him to extend the area of the self-applied massage, but again, it will be useful only to the extent that it is carried out in strict accordance with instructions.

OXYGENATOR, RADIUM AND SALT BATHS (31, 32)

Since the discovery of radio-activity and the many effects which the presence of radium in certain waters and minerals produces on the human body, it has been the special task of research to find means of giving humanity in general the benefit of this important discovery.

The radium preparation, called "Oxygenator," possesses the quality of oxidizing about five times as quickly as any other known substance, and thus removing the degenerated and diseased cells of the human body accordingly.

This material itself, as well as other combinations of radio products and salts I use and prescribe for half or whole baths, as the case may require.

They are of the greatest assistance in carrying out the course of treatment in each individual case. What in former times could be effected only through expensive trips to the few famous healing springs of the world, can now be accomplished in the comfort of the home or the sanatorium. But these measures, too, should be followed only in strict accordance with the physician's orders, bearing in mind that there is such a thing as "too much" even of so valuable an energizer as this.

THE DISEASES TO BE TREATED AND THE APPLICATION OF THE METHOD.

Having given, in the foregoing paragraphs, a brief description of the course of healing which I advocate, I am now about to give a short explanation of the different methods to be applied in treating various forms of disease, all of which have been already explained as degenerations of the twelve tissues of the body. This will enable patients to apply the prescriptions given to their individual cases.

...Once more, however, I warn every one not to commit the mistake of believing that a layman can cure his own disease by even the most careful study of a book such as this is.

To the patient, who has been led into the path of health, it will, as is its purpose, give such instructions as will enable him to see his condition plainly. *He will then be able the more effectively to follow the instructions of the physician, and – what is of equal importance – to inform him correctly in regard to his own observations of his condition and the changes brought about by the treatment.*

There is another point that I wish to mention here at the outset.

Disease, although reduced to its last analysis under this system, is never so simple that it can be determined as the degeneration of one tissue exclusively. The unity of the body, the close connection of the various tissues, and the gradual transition from one into another, make it impossible to draw the lines as sharply and distinctly as between chemical elements. For the sake of classification we make the degeneration of a certain tissue the distinguishing element between various forms of disease. Let us not forget, however, that this does not mean more than the *degeneration of the main tissue* which is affected by this particular complaint, while the same is also characterized by simultaneous degeneration of one or more of the other tissues, only to a lesser degree. It is, therefore, not inconsistent if, in giving the more detailed description thereof, several tissues are mentioned as being degenerated, and not only the one particular tissue from which the class derives its name.

I. DEGENERATION OF THE PLASMO TISSUE.

Anaemia, Chlorosis, Pernicious Anaemia.
A. Scrofulosis. B. Tuberculosis. C. Syphilis. D. Cancer.

To many who are unfamiliar with the results of modern research, and even to many physicians of the old school of medicine, the family of disease forms, as enumerated above, will look somewhat formidable. It comprises the most disastrous plagues of mankind,— plagues for which cures have been so frantically sought with such an ominous lack of results. It thus constitutes one of the most practical revelations of the biological method of research to positively proclaim that the common cause of these manifestly so different constitutional diseases is one and the same.

That this fact was not recognized long ago is the reason they have been pronounced incurable by so many physicians who, by poisoning symptoms, established only a semblance of cure, until biological study led to the recognition of the truth. It discovered that all of these constitutional diseases are essentially blood defects and degenerations, resulting in the destruction of the body tissue in general,— the necessary and logical consequence of an imperfect condition of the blood.

So there is a ray of hope for humanity breaking through the night of despair; that is, that its worst foes can be made to disappear in due time by attack directed at their common root.

Not the knife of the surgeon, not the poison of the physician of the old school, but simply harmonizing the individual life with the laws of nature, will eradicate the cause.

The tremendous importance of the subject, the wide field to be covered, makes it wellnigh impossible to treat the matter within the present limits as extensively as it should be treated. A large part of my book, "Dare To Be Healthy," of which this is but an abstract, deals exhaustively with this topic. There the reader will find the most interesting details in regard to the connection between these widely divergent forms of disease. Their nature as blood-diseases carries with it the fact that they are preeminently persistent through many generations, so that today there is but a minority of human beings in whom all tendency towards them is missing. So predisposition advances with the continuity of environment, the one point at which, at least in the case of the so-called white plague, or tuberculosis, an effort against it has been made.

The development towards the eradication of these evils has been neutralised by the overwhelming importance science has given to the theory of the bacillus as the incentive element of disease, while it is only a product of the same.

The serum and anti-toxin therapy, which in its fight against the bacillus, lost sight of the first task of medicine, that of fighting the disease, was the logical consequence thereof.

The blood liquid which consists of the plasma and red and white blood corpuscles, and is the carrier of the lymph to such parts of the body as are not fed directly by the lymphatic vessels, such as the nerves, must have a well defined chemical composition in order to fulfil its task. What we call deficiency of blood is, with the exception of traumatically inflicted losses, normal in quantity, to a great extent, but deficient in quality. This consists in the chemical composition and the proportion of nutritive salts in the serum, or in the relation and quality of the oxygen carriers, that is, the red and white corpuscles, whose task it is to remove foreign and disturbing elements from the blood.

It is obvious that deficiency in these elements may be of infinite variety and of the most far reaching consequence for the various tissues of the body, which receive their nourishment therefrom.

According to the nature of the effects which this variety in blood deficiency (dysaemia) produces, we distinguish certain groups of degenerations in the body, for which names were established at a time when the unity of these forms of disease had not yet been recognized. Thus, where dysaemia produces only general debility, we call it anaemia, which may gradually become destructive and develop into "pernicious" anaemia. When it affects girls with all kinds of disturbances in menstruation, perverting their appetite and causing a greenish color of the skin, it is called "chlorosis." If the symptoms are the destruction of the lymphatic glands, so often noticed in children said to be hereditarily affected, we speak of "Scrofulosis." When erroneous composition of the blood, produced by poor living and unsanitary environment, causes destruction of the lungs or of certain bones or tissues, the name "tuberculosis" indicates that the decaying condition of the affected tissues results in producing numerous tubercle bacilli. In the many cases in which the destruction is even more widespread, attacking the skin, bones, brain and other tissues or organs, and where the decomposing poison, if not hereditary, has entered the blood by way of sexual intercourse, the ominous word "syphilis" indicates the resulting blood disease. When the weakened tissues, which are not sufficiently fed with the elements they need for their normal existence, cannot resist the developing power of the phosphates prevalent in the blood, the much dreaded malign "cancer growths" appear.

The destructions wrought by dysaemia in these various forms, cannot be fully described in this brief abstract. They can all be reduced, arrested and forced to give place to healthy regeneration by the hygienic-dietetic healing system. In each case, however, the possibility of cure will depend entirely on the degree of decomposition which has been reached. If the trouble is from hereditary tendency it is obviously harder to fight, and a long regenerative treatment may be anticipated. If attacked at an early stage, complete restoration to health is possible in a comparatively short period.

The most careful and thorough investigation by the physician must precede any treatment. It is his task to prescribe accordingly, with the development of the disease and its gradual disappearance.

The simultaneous direct and indirect affection of various tissues, especially of the lymphatics, will necessitate more complicated application of the various nutritive compositions.

THERAPY.

Diet: I. For the Anaemic.

All that grows in the sunshine makes blood. Therefore, the food of an anaemic person should consist mainly of articles of diet which grow above the surface, such as green vegetables, fresh greens, fruit, berries. Since the blood has already grown very thin, as little fluid as possible should be taken, and for this reason the boasted milk cures are far from advisable. If all hot reasoning is avoided and little salt and sugar are used, no thirst will be felt. Coffee, tea, beer, wine and other alcoholic drinks are to be avoided because they consume oxygen, such as also do thin soups, lemonade, malt coffee, and other beverages of slight food value.

Breakfast: In summer, a glass of cold milk, sweet or sour, and with it strawberries, huckleberries, cherries, or other fruit in season; in winter milk or cocoa, oatmeal porridge with bread (whole wheat, whole rye), or something similar. When the bowels are sluggish, take a little fruit on rising in the morning and at bedtime.

Dinner: Cereals, rice, macaroni, dumplings and eggs, with fresh greens, spinach, fresh peas, fresh beans, cauliflower, all varieties of cabbage, cucumbers, pumpkins and squashes. Root vegetables are not excluded. Celery and parsnips alone interfere with the renewal of blood. They ought not to be eaten frequently.

Afternoon Lunch: Fruit, milk or one cup only of weak cocoa. If the appetite is good, omit this meal.

Supper: Every day, if possible, some fresh greens seasoned with lemon juice, particularly cresses, lettuce, endive, spinach and red cabbage, with puddings of meal or eggs. Sour milk with fruit and mild cheese, may be taken for a change. In winter, thick soup or porridge with fruit, preferably apples and huckleberries. Also an apple at bedtime.

Anaemic people commonly have no wish for meat. They force themselves to eat it in the belief that only on a meat diet is it possible for them to become strong. They would do better to follow their inclination and refrain from it altogether. They regain health faster on a purely vegetable diet, one special reason being that the digestion is less burdened.

Fattening, combined with rest and rational remedies, like Dech-Manna-Diet, are the best means of curing anaemia.

The deficient appetite must be stimulated through tastefully prepared dishes and much variety. The patient will thus unconsciously be induced to take more food. Delicacies and dainty dishes foster pleasure in eating, and a little food between the principal meals will help to make up the necessary amount. Spinach, also egg omelettes filled with spinach, puddings, groat, oatmeal, light dishes prepared with plenty of eggs, sugar, butter and milk, also roasted meat if desired are the best articles of food for anaemic patients. Drinks that are recommended are: strong malt extracts, buttermilk, sour milk, Dech-Manna chocolate, fruit coffees, fruits, berries, honey and Dech-Manna-Diet.

I. and II. A. For Scrofulous Patients.

Two affections, rachitis and scrofula, frequently co-exist, and the same dietary is appropriate for both. Scrofulous patients often have a great longing for sulphur and for irritating compounds. Frequently they consume salt greedily, eat charcoal, onions, and other piquant substances. This indicates their need of vegetables and fresh greens full of nutritious salts and of pungent taste and smell because of the amount of sulphur they contain.

Various kinds of cabbage are appropriate for the principal dinner dish, cooked or raw in the form of a salad, with horseradish to give them relish. For seasoning of vegetables and salads, onions and leeks may be used unsparingly; onion soups will be found palatable and will improve the lymph.

At supper water-cress, lettuce, radishes, and sandwiches made of chives are preferable to sausage and rich cheese. Fresh, mild cheese makes a good side-dish.

Meat should be eaten sparingly, because it rapidly changes into products of decomposition in the lymph, and so the harmful rather than the useful fluids of the body are increased.

In connection with rachitis and scrofula a ravenous appetite is often manifested. This is a morbid symptom. It arises from exhaustion of the stomach and intestines, for no increase of bodily weight accompanies it. The greater part of the nourishment taken passes out of the system without being digested. Such persons, whether adults or children, should have their meals at regular, short intervals, for they are unable to restrain their morbid eagerness for food. After a few days of strict diet they lose their appetite, a condition that must be accepted until a natural hunger takes its place and results in a normal increase in bodily weight.

It is well known that many people suffer from hives and eczema after having eaten certain dishes, such as crawfish, strawberries, oysters, honey, tomatoes or cheese. For such people to refrain from partaking of this kind of food is no protection against eczema. Only regeneration of the blood will lead to a cure.

As a rule such patients should avoid sharp and spicy dishes; especially desirable is a diet of fresh, good meat, not in very large quantity, alternating with days on which no meat at all is taken. It is imperative to avoid sharp cheese, such as Roquefort, mustard, sardelles, mixed pickles and similar spicy dishes. Form VI is best for patients suffering from scrofulosis.

I. and II. B. For Tuberculosis Patients.

Patients who suffer from diseases of the lungs or other tubercular tissues do not require food of different composition than is generally recommended, provided their digestive organs are healthy. They must have albumen (medium fat beef, veal lean pork, haddie, pickled herring, eggs, brick cheese, peas) and fat in sufficient, even abundant quantity. Warmed milk is recommended especially. Variety in food should prevail. This will be the best means of overcoming the dangerous lack of appetite, which must be stimulated by delicacies and cleverly prepared dishes given between meals, sandwiches, cold fowl, jellies, piquant cold meats. The single portions should be small but frequent. Good beer rich in malt, sherry, malaga and other sweet wines, are all able to promote the appetite, unless the physician orders strict abstinence from alcohol.

In case of haemorrhage of the lungs, the physician will generally prescribe liquid food exclusively, and his orders must be observed strictly. In such cases it is very advisable to take gelatine, which can be prepared in a variety of ways, or meat jellies.

Care should be taken in all forms of tubercular patients, that the special tissue gets its special composition.

I. and II. C. For Syphilitic Patients.

The diet for people affected with syphilis does not vary from the one given under I and II. A. for scrofulous patients. Just as in the case of scrofulosis, a rich diet is recommended for syphilis. (Form VI).

In former times starvation-cures were applied in case of syphilis, based on the hypothesis that diseased humours in the body should be reduced. In view of the noxious effect which the disease exercises on the entire body, this method has been given up. In case of the hereditary syphilis of infants, the best possible diet for the mother must always be insisted upon. (Never less than Form VI and Dech-Manna Eubiogen, with each meal). If nursing by the mother is impossible, and since a wet-nurse cannot be subjected to the danger of contamination through the child, easily digestible substitutes for mother's milk should be selected; that is, not cow's milk, but other approved nutritive foods for infants. It will be most beneficial to add Dech-Manna Eubiogen Liquid to the child's food.

I. and II. D. For Cancer Patients.

Cachectic patients should not, as some authorities recommended in former times, be starved by poor diet in addition to the losses which they already suffer when afflicted with diseases, such as cancer. Except in case of cancer of the stomach and bowels, when I would recommend Form III and, with gradual improvement, an increase up to Form VI, the latter form of diet should always be prescribed in case of cancer. Special instructions, as given under the heading, I. and II. C. For Syphilitic Patients, should also be followed in these cases.

Dech-Manna-Compositions:

(Only main compositions, specialities to Doctor's order).
I. Anaemia: Plasmogen, Eubiogen.
I. and II. A. Scrofulosis: Plasmogen, Lymphogen, Dermogen, Eubiogen.

I. and II. B. Tuberculosis: **Plasmogen**, **Lymphogen**, Mucogen, Gelatinogen, **Eubiogen**

I. and II. C. Syphilis: **Plasmogen**, **Lymphogen**, Dermogen, **Eubiogen**

I. and II. D. Cancer: **Plasmogen**, **Lymphogen**, **Eubiogen.**

Physical:

I. Anaemia. Breathing Exercises.

I. and II. A. Scrofulosis: Partial Packs, Oxygenator baths, Radium and
Salt whole baths.

I. and II. B. Tuberculosis: Ablutions, Breathing Exercises.

I. and II. C. Syphilis Abdominal packs, Partial packs, Oxygenator, Radium
and Salt half baths.

I. and II. D. Cancer: Oxygenator, Radium and Salt whole baths.

II. DEGENERATION OF THE LYMPH TISSUE.

The lymph, the second life-giving fluid, is first drawn from the chyle, the milky juice, into which all food is converted after it leaves the stomach, and after having directly fed the nerves, enters the blood through the ductus thoracicus, and accompanies it in its circulation.

According to its nature some degenerations of the lymph tissue are coincident with degenerations of the blood, and especially the plasma, such as Scrofulosis, Tuberculosis, Syphilis and Cancer, while other degenerations of the lymph tissue coincide with degenerations of the lymph-fed nerve tissue and are consequently treated under that heading.

III. DEGENERATION OF THE NERVE TISSUE.

The nerves which form the very complicated system of gelatinous cords of various sizes which emanate from the brain and the spinal cord, send thousands of branches throughout the entire body. They communicate the impressions from the outside to the brain and convey its conscious or unconscious (instinctive) mandate to the muscles of all organs.

The nerves are fed by the lymphatic system and are everywhere accompanied by blood-vessles, and the oxygenous blood in the latter conveys the oxygen to the nerve substance, which it consumes and thus develops power sufficient to execute the various functions.

Naturally the supply that replaces the burned nerve substance, must be adequate, and if for any reason whatsoever more nerve substance is consumed than the body is able to renew by the time it is needed, the nerve system becomes degenerated and numerous disturbances are the consequence.

This is the great field of mental functions and disturbances, of moods and reactions on muscular tracts which in themselves are healthy, but are paralyzed in their work through the defective functioning of the power-conveying nerves.

Again it is impossible here to give more than a general description, showing on what conditions nervous diseases are based. The manifold manifestations of this degeneration were combined into groups under the old system in which the Greek name of a system was everything, its practical explanation but little.

The principal ways in which these degenerations manifest themselves are pains, mental agony and derangement, temporary cessation of functions, cramps, involuntary movements and similar disturbances.

The names generally applied to them are neuralgia and neuritis,—causing pains in the nerves of certain parts of the body; neurasthenia,—consisting mainly of the complete relaxation of tension in the nervous system, causing sadness, inability for work, etc.; asthma, cramp-like cessation of certain functions of the small vessels of the lungs, alveoli, which impedes respiration; epilepsy, temporary cramp in the greater part of the body, causing loss of consciousness, involuntary movements of the limbs, etc.; St. Vitus's dance, — a similar affection, usually in children.

While the complicated nature of nerve diseases requires very careful treatment of great individual variety, the general rule is that the re-enforcement of the nerves with the material of which they are built, together with regeneration of the blood, which, when in normal condition prevents such disturbances, will bring about a cure. Of course this is sometimes a slow process, especially when, as in the case of epilepsy, the nervous disease is of an hereditary character, and the resistant power of the nerves is correspondingly weak.

In regard to one of the most disastrous diseases, caused by degeneration of the most important nerve i.e. the Vagus, see under "Catarrh" — section VI.

THERAPY.

Diet: If the entire nervous system is in a condition of pathological irritability, as in cases of neurasthenia and hysteria, it is the object of rational diet to keep all irritations from such a vibrating organism.

To prescribe: "No coffee, no tea, no alcohol, no strong spices and no tobacco," will do no harm, and in most cases will prove beneficial.

Nothing is more absurd than the attempt to strengthen nervous people by the use of alcohol. When forbidden alcohol entirely, it will very often transpire that some symptom, like headache, neuralgia, etc., was due to its use. Whenever the general conditions permit the continued use of alcohol to a certain extent, it must not be left to the patient's judgment to determine how far this may go, but definite quantities must be prescribed in each individual case, although the patient's experience may be of assistance in determining the quantity. (Moritz).

Good results have been obtained by limiting the meat diet of extremely nervous patients, and prescribing for them a diet consisting principally of milk, eggs, cereals, vegetables and fruits. In this way the irritating effect of many of the meat extracts is avoided. At the same time the digestive work of the stomach, reduced by the limited meat diet, and the stimulation of stool, always promoted by a prevalence of vegetable elements in the diet, exercises a beneficial influence on the condition of the patient.

Disturbances of the stomach and intestines are very closely connected with neurasthenia, loss of strength of the nerve-tissue, and hysteria, in some cases being the cause, and in other cases, which occur more frequently, the consequence of the same.

Excessive and, more rarely, defective secretion of hydrochloric acid by the stomach cells, cramps, general atony or debility, of the stomach, vomiting, diarrhoea, constipation, tympanites (excessive production of gases), may all arise from nervous causes. In such cases the diet must be the same as given for nervous disease.

Not only in these cases, but in most instances of nervous diseases, a diet which does not produce irritation and excludes alcohol, will have to be prescribed. The danger of alcohol in cases of peripheric neuritis, epilepsy and mental diseases, is obvious.

Epileptics, like other nervous patients, should receive a diet that is mainly, but not solely, a vegetable diet, exclusive of all highly spiced food.

The same principles govern in case of Basedow's disease, which is a special type of irritating disease.

Absolutely necessary foodstuffs to be recommended in this case are clams, sole and water cress, because they contain more organic iodine than any other known food-stuff.

As iodine is the basic mineral of the thyroid gland, and other preparations are poisonous or dangerous, the necessity of partaking of these dishes becomes obvious, in addition to the fact that if properly prepared, they are delicious. This organic iodine will regulate the secretions of the glands.

A diet void of irritation is also most important for children who suffer from nervous conditions, such as St. Vitus's dance, involuntary urination during sleep, etc. Alcohol and alkaline and carbonated drinks must also be avoided in all nervous conditions that are combined with hyperaemia of the brain, as meningitis, apoplexia, tumors of the brain, etc., since they produce congestions.

Special dietetic directions cannot be given for all of the innumerable varieties of the various other nervous complaints. The general principle must always govern, that sufficient food is the natural foundation, not only of the self-healing tendencies of the organism, but also of any effective therapy.

In special cases where neurasthenia and hysteria or nervous dyspepsia prevail, it will be necessary to apply a special diet to be prescribed by the physician, who must understand the underlying cause, which is, 9 times out of ten, the degeneration of the Vagus nerve. See article on Influenza.

DECH-MANNA-COMPOSITIONS
(Only main compositions, specialities to Doctor's order)

Acute form, Neuralgia, Neuritis: **Neurogen**, Plasmogen, Eubiogen.

Chronic form, Asthma, Epilepsy, St. Vitus's Dance: **Neurogen**, Plasmogen, Lymphogen, Eubiogen.

Physical:

Acute form: Partial packs.

Chronic form: Partial packs, Massage

IV. DEGENERATION OF THE BONE TISSUE.

Rickets, Osteomalacia and similar diseases.

The condition of the skeleton,—the solid structure of the osseous frame,—is of the greatest importance to the maintenance of health. Its various forms of disease,—such as deficient development of bone; osteomalacia,—softening of the bones; flat foot; caries—molecular decay or death of the bones, especially of the teeth,—are based mostly upon rachitis (rickets).

Rachitis should be fought at the time the child develops in the womb, by properly feeding the mother and preparing her to give it, after birth, healthy milk, with all the elements necessary for bone structure.

Rachitis is principally lack of lime in the food, which causes parts of the bones to remain soft instead of becoming rigid.

It is a constitutional, often hereditary, disease caused by poor nutrition and by influences of environment, such as marshy regions and humid climates.

The lack of lime in the food is often obvious when children show a tendency to eat chalk, and even to scratch walls in order to eat the lime obtained therefrom.

More solid food, that gives work to the teeth and the digestive organs, is certainly advisable in such cases.

The symptoms of rachitis become apparent at the pelvis and at the wide open, soft parts of the skull, the unossified fontanelles. The cartilage in the wrists and ankles becomes thick. Slow development of the teeth, swollen glands in the neck, inflammations in different parts of the body, cramps and convulsions,—among others, of the vocal cords,—are further indications. In the progressive development of the disease, the softened cartilage grows and protrudes everywhere, especially in the thorax, such as "rachitis rosary." Crooked bones and hunchbacks not infrequently develop.

Therapy.

Diet: Older children should receive chopped meat, eggs, zwieback or whole grain bread. Bouillon will stimulate their digestion. Uffelmann recommends a mixture of one part veal bouillon and two to three parts of milk, which children like.

It is unnecessary to give calcium directly, when a rachitic diet is observed. Sufficient is contained in the Dech-Manna-Diet, given principally in milk and as a rule also in the drinking water.

Quantities of amylaceous (starchy) food, candy, cakes and other sweets, coarse vegetables and potatoes must be avoided, since with children they are the cause of stomach trouble, resulting in decomposition and the formation of acids in the intestines.

Breakfast: Milk and whole grain bread, or oatmeal porridge and fruit.—Whole grain bread signifies any variety of bread made from flour containing the entire contents of the grain, the gluten as well as the bran; among these are Graham-bread, rye-bread, pilot-bread, and Rhenish black bread.

Mid-morning Lunch: Raw scraped carrots; for small children and for those having poor teeth, oat flakes.

Dinner: Every other day—legumes, prepared in various ways, and fruit, vegetables or fresh greens; for example:

(a) White beans boiled to the consistency of a thick soup, with apples.

(b) Fresh pea soup containing rice, barley, sweet corn or oatmeal; a thick pea-porridge with parsley, served with carrots, cabbage, white turnips, red cabbage, Savoy cabbage, or various fresh greens; or simply browned.

(c) Dried pea soup with similar contents; barley porridge, fresh greens, baked potatoes; or browned and eaten with any vegetables.

(d) Lentils boiled in soup with the same contents as before; or as porridge, particularly with potatoes and fresh greens.

Care must be taken never to eat leguminous products in large quantities, because their nutritious properties are so high. Potatoes should be used whole when added to other vegetables, and steamed not strained, because they easily lose thereby their valuable sulphuric contents.

Afternoon Lunch: Fruit and whole grain bread, or a glass of milk and bread.

Supper: In summer, cold or warm porridge with fruit and fresh greens, and besides these millet, buckwheat, oats, barley and Graham-bread, as especially efficient bone material. Sweet or sour milk proves a relishing addition. In winter, soup made of the above grains, or of potatoes not deprived of their mineral contents by peeling and straining.

Dech-Manna-Compositions: **Osseogen**, Plasmogen, Cartillogen, Eubiogen.

Physical: Gymnastics, Massage.

V. DEGENERATION OF THE MUSCULAR TISSUE.

Muscular Rheumatism, Sciatica, Infantile Paralysis, Atrophy, Amyloid Organs.

The muscles, about 400 pairs, which must perform all the actual work of the body, require good nourishment through the blood, which will rapidly replace the cells that are constantly used up.

Muscular degeneration is caused by disturbances in the quality and circulation of the blood.

Interruption in the proper circulation of the blood, stagnation etc., cause *rheumatism* with intense pains, and this can be removed only by restoring the undisturbed circulation of the blood, carrying all substances requisite for the proper nutrition of the muscles.

If disease of the muscular tissue combines with a diseased condition of the accompanying nerves, we speak of *Sciatica*.

Infantile paralysis, which often appears suddenly, muscular atrophy, which develops slowly, *progressive and chronic atrophy* of the muscles, are also forms of muscular disease, combined with destruction of the accompanying nerve tissue.

A special group of muscular diseases consists of amyloid (fatty) degeneration of vital muscle substance, as for instance of the heart, the kidneys, the liver. These are also caused by faulty composition of the blood, which does not feed the muscles with the substances required and thus causes them to degenerate by developing too much fat.

The predisposition for such forms of disease is very often inherited.

Amyloid degeneration is often combined with wasting diseases, such as atrophy, tuberculosis and dropsy.

Therapy.

Diet: Sufferers from gout must always be guided by the necessity of avoiding all food that contains large quantities of acid. In a general way it is also necessary to live moderately in every respect and so avoid all excesses.

There are a number of dishes that are harmful to such patients. Among them are various meats, especially dark roast meat, also game. In general, and especially in very severe cases, it is better to refrain from white meat also. Spleen, liver, kidney, sweetbread, brains are absolutely prohibited, also sausage and smoked and canned meats, oily fish, especially eel, salmon, pike, and all smoked fish, because they may create a large amount of uric acid.

The amount of meat eaten must not exceed 200 grams per day. The following must also be avoided: all sharp cheeses, cabbage, sauerkraut, and beans.

Among vegetables the following are recommended: asparagus, celery and potatoes. The vegetables containing oxalic acid, such as spinach, sorrel, rhubarb and cress it is best to avoid.

Butter is permitted in small quantities, also eggs.

Sweet farinose dishes are unnecessary.

Tea and coffee are allowed as beverages in very small amounts. The principal drinks, however, should be mineral waters, such as Vichy, Apollinaris, etc., which may be varied from time to lime.

It is strongly recommended that the patients eat much fruit. Fruit-acids promote good circulation.

Breakfast: (a) In winter, tea made from the leaves of the haw, blackberry, or strawberry, cereal coffee, weak cocoa with bread and butter.

(b) In summer, sour milk, fruit juices, or fruit and bread; among fruits particularly strawberries, currants, gooseberries, huckleberries, cherries, grapes, apples.

Mid-morning Lunch: Radishes mashed with apples, also a raw cucumber or tomato in the form of a salad.

Dinner: No meat, no soup; fresh greens, fresh vegetables with potatoes, rice, macaroni, and a dish of corn, rice, groats, peas, beans, tomatoes or mushrooms. In addition, light custard with fruit or sweetmeats with fruit.

Afternoon Lunch: Fruit only.

Supper: Fresh lettuce, with macaroni, baked potatoes, pancakes, custard; or radishes with cream and potatoes, custard, mild cheese and leeks.

Exclusive fruit dietaries, comprising strawberries, currants, cherries and grapes, are effective in preventing eruptions on the skin and removing their effects.

From one to three-quarters of a pound of fruit should be eaten at a meal, either with a little bread or with sour milk, and at dinner as a desert.

In winter, from three to seven lemons a day serve the same purpose. The juice is used without sugar and with as little water as possible, never with the meal, but a little before, or in the morning on an empty stomach. Only fresh lemons should be used for this purpose, not the prepared lemon juice which is on the market. Tomatoes may be eaten in the raw state, likewise.

In mild cases of gout and rheumatism some crisp lean meat and fish may be eaten, but not every day. A diet without meat has a better curative effect upon the disease.

Alcohol is to be shunned as totally inadmissible. The wines which contain no alcohol must serve as substitutes.

Special Diet: For Diseases of the Heart and Inactive Kidneys.

Patients, who are afflicted with any kind of heart or kidney disease, must be very careful never to overload the stomach. They should eat small meals, at frequent intervals, and avoid irritating food; the amount of liquids and milk must be determined by the physician. A moderate amount of salt only is allowed, and if the physician so prescribes, a diet containing little salt, must be observed.

In case of acute inflammation of the kidneys, meat is absolutely prohibited; the best diet is an exclusive milk-diet, consisting of at least 1 to 1½ quarts fresh milk, and in certain cases warmed milk, taken by the spoonful; the quantity to be increased, if necessary, to 3 and 4 quarts per day. Instead of milk, buttermilk, sour milk, kefir, koumiss or yoghurt may be taken.

Beef broths are strictly prohibited. In their place glutenous soups, of oats, barley sago, tapioca, rice, groat, may be taken; furthermore leguminos soups, made from the preparations of the firms Knorr, Liebig, Maggi, and others. 1 to 2 spoonfuls of these preparations are put into a cupful of water, some salt is added and the mixture is then boiled.

A more varied diet is allowed in lighter forms of the disease, such as milk dishes, mashed potatoes, preserved apples or pears, rolls and butter, bread, cream, cream cheese, farinaceous dishes, eggs and green vegetables, meat according to the orders of the physician. Spices and alcohol must be strictly avoided.

In cases of chronic kidney diseases, greater variety should be observed in the diet. In any event, however, a certain quantity of milk should be taken, not less than 1 quart per day.

The following food is to be limited: All game, including birds, sausages and smoked meat, sweetbread, brains, liver, spleen, crawfish, lobster, rich cheese especially Roquefort, Parmesan, Camembert, all sharp spices, such as pepper, paprika, mustard, cinnamon, garlic, onions; among vegetables such as radishes, horseradish, celery asparagus, mushrooms, tomatoes, sorrel; furthermore, all meat extracts, piquant sauces and soup spices.

No alcohol should be served on the table of a patient with kidney disease. The exceptions must be prescribed by the physician. The same applies to all new wines and beef soups.

The following dishes are permitted: Among meats, white meat (about 200 grams per day, preferably at noon). This comprises domestic fowl, fresh pork, lamb and veal, also beef, especially boiled beef. As a variety from time to time, mutton and fresh fish.

The preferable way to prepare dishes for patients suffering from kidney diseases, is to boil them; the next best way is to steam them, and the third and least desirable way is frying.

Strongly recommended: calf's feet and pig's feet, calf's head, especially in the form of jellies and pickled, if so ordered by the physician. Occasionally raw beef may be given, but without sharp spices.

Fish: Trout, pike, carp; Saltwater fish: haddock and cod-fish, boiled blue; also frogs' legs. Eggs are permitted, soft boiled, 2 to 3 per day.

Vegetables: With the exception of those mentioned, vegetables are very commendable, especially potatoes, green peas, white and yellow turnips, red beets, cauliflower, lentils, beans, the last particularly, mashed; also salad with cream and a little mild vinegar or lemon juice. Fruit-acids must not be classified with vegetable or meat-acids, as several, so-called "Food-Specialists" try to impress on patients, for they do not know, what they talk about.

Fats, such as cream, butter, rich cheese, olive oil, may be given if they agree with the patient; bacon is not so good.

Bread, white as well as brown, and especially Graham bread, may be eaten without restrictions.

As drinks: mineral water with lemon or orange juice added. Raspberry juice is permitted, but currant and gooseberry juice must be avoided on account of the substances contained in them irritating to the kidneys. Fruit juices free from alcohol (apple cider) may be given.

Every *morning* on rising, a glass of fruit juice or some fruit. These fruit-acids promote peristaltics of the bowels, and free circulation of the blood.

At *supper*: Salad of cresses or celery, or a mixed salad, radishes, asparagus, squash and cucumbers.

When the urinary flows is very scanty, supper may consist of a cup of celery soup, or asparagus broth; in winter, haw tea.

A few suggestions for *dinner*, omitting meat entirely:

Dumplings with cabbage salad, red cabbage or Bavarian cabbage; sliced oatmeal cake with fruit.—Cucumbers with eggs and potato bread, rolled griddle cakes and fruit.—Cabbage with rice and butter, griddle cakes with fresh greens.

Squash with lemon, potatoes, baked beans, fruit.—Red cabbage with macaroni, potato fritters, with fruit.—Dumplings and pears, lettuce.—White turnips with cream and potatoes, buckwheat groats, fruit.—Pea soup with sweet corn, squash and rice with fruit.—Lentils and potatoes, salad of celery or beets, fruit.—Asparagus with drawn butter and parsley sauce and bread dumplings, oat groats with fruit.—Cauliflower with macaroni, buckwheat groats and milk.—Cabbage with browned potatoes, oatmeal cake with fruit.

For Irritable Kidneys (Inflammation, Supperation, Contraction, etc.), and Diseases of the Bladder.

For patients suffering from these diseases all spiced and sharp dishes are prohibited, especially dishes with much pepper and mustard, also mixed pickles, preserves containing vinegar, salads unless seasoned with lemon juice instead of vinegar; furthermore, dishes which produce gas, such as dishes made from yeast. Fruits are permitted only in small quantities, avoiding absolutely gooseberries and preserves made from the same. Preserves from other fruits, such as apples and cherries, are permitted in smaller quantities.

As drinks, the mineral waters which are recommended for people suffering from gout, are advisable here also.

Kidney stones require a mixed diet, preferably vegetable; fat and carbohydrates—very little meat—no sweetbread, kidneys, brains, liver or spleen; meat, if taken at all, must be boiled.

Not permitted: game, pickled fish, piquant sauces, beef broth.

Dispense with meat, raw celery, radishes, pears, cucumbers, even asparagus in large amounts, at least during the state of inflammation. Eat eggs only in a raw or very soft boiled state. In place of these foods make up a diet of milk preparations, rice, groats, oats, millet, buckwheat. Currant juice and wild cherries, apple sauce, diluted lemon juice, are all of great benefit. Soups made from squash, cucumbers or celery, haw tea, buttermilk and sour milk, mild cheese, or porridge and fruit are excellent supper dishes.

For Liver Disease.

In general, fatty substances should be eliminated as much as possible from the nourishment in the case of liver disease, jaundice and gall stones.

To be recommended are light farinaceous dishes with milk, vegetables, fruit and all easily digestible foods.

Meat must be taken only in very small quantities, according to the advice of the physician, and with very little fat. Spices and alcohol are prohibited. Pastry and rich foods must be avoided.

In case of jaundice the patient should receive liquid food only during the first few days, consisting of soups, light tea, carbonated waters; later, milk, the yolks of eggs, zwieback and light milk dishes.

Patients suffering from gall stones may receive the same diet as prescribed for those suffering from liver disease, generally speaking.

In case of liver disease it is necessary to adhere very strictly to the prescriptions of the physician, since they are due to various reasons, and only the physician can give the proper individual directions, after having determined the cause.

Every morning on rising, a glass of unsweetened lemonade, or a wineglass of currant wine or grape juice, or some acid fruit. — The same on retiring at night.

For a second breakfast, four or six radishes, or a tablespoonful of grated radish, or a teaspoonful of horseradish mixed with broth and white bread, eaten with a little toast and butter. — The same for supper.

The following are a few suggestions for dinner without meat:

Cabbage, potato porridge, gooseberries with egg and milk sauce. — Lentils with potatoes and fresh greens, cresses or lettuce, fruit. — Savoy cabbage with rice and tomato sauce, fruit with millet cakes. — Leeks with potatoes, macaroni and plums. — Young green beans with dried white beans and apples or other fruit, beets with cream, rolled dumplings, fruits. — White cabbage with macaroni, chopped apples or curdled milk.

Dech-Manna Compositions: (Only main compositions, specialities to the Doctor's order.)

Rheumatism: **Muscogen**, **Plasmogen**, Eubiogen.

Sciatica: **Muscogen**, **Plasmogen**, Neurogen, Eubiogen.

Amyloid heart: **Muscogen**, **Plasmogen**, Eubiogen.

Amyloid kidney or liver: **Muscogen**, **Plasmogen**, Mucogen, Eubiogen.

Physical: Rheumatism: Partial packs, either vinegar and water or radium and salts. Massage, if necessary, and special oxygenator baths, and radium and salt baths.

Sciatica: Leg packs, oxygenator baths, half radium and salt baths, followed by massage.

Amyloid heart, kidney or liver: Abdominal packs, gymnastics, oxygenator baths, whole radium and salt baths.

VI. DEGENERATION OF THE MUCOUS MEMBRANE TISSUE.

Catarrh in acute and chronic forms, bronchitis, pleurisy, pneumonia, inflammation of nose, throat, bowels, stomach, bladder.

Decomposition of mucous membrane, hemorrhoids, polyps, benign tumors, also Bright's disease in initial stages.

Catarrhal disease is amongst the most common, in varied form and degree, owing to the very tender nature of the mucous membrane.

These ailments are characterized as destructions of the protective membranes which cover the serous layer of the organs, in which layer the lymph circulates.

The numerous ends of blood-vessels and nerves which are thus exposed to attack, and the spreading of the disease to healthy tissues which thus become affected in the same way, make the various catarrhal troubles with their accompanying excretions particularly unpleasant.

All degenerations of the mucous membrane are based on deficiencies in blood circulation and composition.

A cure is effected through the restoration of the serous layer to normal conditions and the regeneration of the blood and its circulation.

These various forms of catarrh affect all parts that are covered with mucous membranes, among them the female sexual organs, hence leukorrhoea or fluor albus, which, if not properly treated, constitutes the basis for all sorts of polyps, tumors, etc., and in many cases of continued attack forms the predisposition to cancer.

The lymphatic system is the carrier of all germs to the various mucous membranes, and promotes the spreading of catarrh to all parts of the body.

Among the more serious and dangerous forms of acute disease of this class which, lacking proper treatment, develop into chronic forms, are the catarrhal affections of the lungs and bronchia, **grippe**, **influenza**, [B] catarrh of the intestines, the bladder, the hemorrhoids and Bright's (kidney) disease. The latter especially is among the most dangerous diseases, and is considered incurable by the adherents of the old medical school. The discovery that it is essentially the same as other catarrhal diseases has, however, established the possibility of complete cure, which has been effected in many, even neglected, cases of long standing, under my present system.

The many varieties of symptoms, all of which are finally reduced by proper treatment of the mucous membranes, it is impossible to cite, in this brief synopsis.

More details concerning this important group will be found, together with the modern explanation of the development of serious disease from apparently unimportant catarrhal affections, in the very complete and extensive descriptions given in Chapter X, Section 6, of my greater work.

Therapy.

Diet: (a) Catarrh in all its acute forms.

In these cases the diet is almost identical with the fever diet, as given in Forms II, III, and IV.

(b) Catarrh in all its chronic forms.

Diet as above, but apply Forms IV, V, VI.

(c) Haemorrhoids, Polyps, Adenoids, Benign Tumors or Fungus Growths.

There are no special prescriptions for these, regarding diet, except that easily digestible food must be eaten. Mashed vegetables and fruit should prevail. The indigestible tissues, such as skin, sinews and gristle, should be removed from the meat. No gas-producing dishes, such as sauerkraut, cabbage, turnips or beans, ought to be taken.

Throat and Larynx Disease.

To avoid irritation of the mucous membranes of the mouth and larynx, all sharp and spicy dishes and drinks are prohibited.

In case of fever, particularly recommended are warm glutenous soups, creams, milk, steamed fruit, fruit soups and sauces, minced white meat, baked or steamed fish, no sharp spices.

Dech-Manna-Compositions: (Only main compositions, specialities to the Doctor's order). In general: **Muscogen**.

Bronchitis, Pleurisy, Pneumonia, Inflammation of nose, throat, bowels, stomach, bladder, also benign growths in all chronic forms. **Muscogen, Plasmogen**, Gelatinogen, Eubiogen.

Bright's disease: (See special section XII chapt. X, "Dare to be healthy.")

Physical Treatment.

Bronchitis, pleurisy: Ablutions with vinegar and water; partial packs or ablutions with vinegar and water; shoulder packs.

Pneumonia: Shoulder packs.

Inflammation of nose, throat etc.: Partial packs or radium and salt three-quarter packs.

Inflammation, of bowels, stomach and bladder: Warm abdominal packs in addition to the above.

Catarrh in chronic forms: Cold abdominal packs, massage.

Decomposition of mucous membrane: Abdominal packs, partial packs, with vinegar and water, or salt and radium emanation, oxygenator and other baths, in case especially prescribed.

VII. DEGENERATION OF TOOTH AND EYE TIS-SUES.

It has been explained that this unusual method of classifying the eyes and the teeth together in one group, is based upon the biological, chemical discovery that the lens of the eye, like the enamel of the teeth, contain fluoric acid, otherwise contained also in very small quantities in the enamel of the finger-and toe-nails.

Disease of the eyes and of the teeth would require lengthy description, for which space is lacking; suffice it to mention that the best way of preserving the health of the teeth and of the eyes is to keep them scrupulously clean. This simple hygienic method, regarding the teeth, will prevent decay.

In all cases where eye trouble concerns the lens, as well as when there is a general disposition to caries in the teeth, the following treatment will produce a curative and preventive effect.

Therapy

Diet: Since most of the disease of the teeth and eyes is merely the consequence of other disease, such as Bright's disease, diabetes, etc., the diet will be in accordance with the main disease, as described. In the treatment of both, rye bread, which contains large quantities of fluoric acid, is highly recommended.

Dech-Manna-Compositions: Teeth: **Dento-Ophthogen**, **Plasmogen**, Osseogen, Eubiogen. *Eyes*: **Dento-Ophthogen**, **Plasmogen**, Gelatinogen, Eubiogen.

Physical: All physical directions according to the main disease of which the tooth and eye disease, is but an accompanying symptom.

VIII. DEGENERATION OF THE HAIR TISSUE.

The hair, though a tissue by itself, is connected with the rest of the body and nourished by the blood, as are all the other tissues, in organic unity.

In the long course of years that mark the progress of the race, it has lost much of its original significance as a body covering against the elements, but even in its present reduced capacity, it is a good and true indicator of certain deficiencies in the blood and in the functions of the body.

Its principal disease manifests itself in loss, through the shrinkage of the little globular terminal, by means of which it is rooted in the skin.

The hair has become an accepted criterion of youth and beauty, and its change in color or its loss are consequently regarded as the unfailing heralds of approaching age. The vast majority of people accept this fact with reluctance, and thus the hair, more than any other feature has become a centre of the nefarious activities of impostors.

Its loss can be prevented to a great extent, and its quality kept in healthy condition, if it is treated in the proper hygienic-dietetic manner.

Therapy.

Diet: Diet in case of hair disease calls for a combination of food containing lime, silica and gelatine. It must be selected from a list of foods that possess these special nourishing qualities.

Dech-Manna-Compositions **Capillogen**, **Plasmogen**, Gelatinogen, Eubiogen.

Physical: No special directions required.

IX. DEGENERATION OF THE SKIN TISSUE.

According to the conception of the human body as a unit, it is not difficult to understand that the skin, while not a separate organ, forms the outermost layer of the body-tissues and is nourished *from within*.

By means of more than 2,500,000 small openings in the skin, called the pores, communication is established between the external and the internal parts of the body. This produces a permanent exchange of matter, and thus the skin is, in fact, a second system of respiration of the greatest importance to the health of the entire body.

Naturally it is subject to traumatic accidents through its exposed position. Traumatic affections cannot now be discussed; except to give a brief idea of the constitutional diseases of the skin which, like all others, originate in deficient blood. Often they are only secondary, and indications of various, more complicated, diseases. In a few cases they affect the skin alone, but are nevertheless constitutional, especially in such cases as could not exist at all, were the disposition not established constitutionally.

There is hardly another department of medicine where the "quack" reaps so great a harvest as in the treatment of skin diseases. Thus the suppression of symptoms becomes the rule; the removal of causes is invariably neglected. Many forms of skin disease, being the result of sexual infections, are allowed to develop because prudery and other motives prevent the early investigation of the cause, and hence delay its prompt treatment and healing.

It is easy and natural for every one to notice the skin and see when there is anything amiss.

Upon discovery immediately consult an hygienic-dietetic physician, and follow his advice closely, since skin diseases are among the most obstinate to overcome. The physician will be able to determine whether there is real constitutional trouble or merely a superficial skin disease. Thus the underlying evil, if any, can be correctly treated, in combination with such specialities as the skin tissue requires.

Every skin disease must be treated from the inside, so as to destroy the disposition and even the chance for development. In view of the large field and the great importance of this group, it will be advisable for every one to read the many pages that have been devoted to this special subject in my work, on "Regeneration" or "Dare To Be Healthy," Chapter X, Section 9.

Therapy.

Diet: The general rule of abstaining from highly seasoned food should govern all patients suffering from skin diseases. Special attention should be given to a diet consisting of good, fresh meat, not too rich; it should be alternated with days on which no meat is eaten. Strong cheese (Roquefort), mustard, sardelles, mixed pickles must be avoided. See also remarks on Scrofulosis under I. A.

Dech-Manna-Compositions: **Dermogen**, **Plasmogen**, Gelatinogen, Eubiogen.

Physical: Partial packs, either vinegar and water, or salt and radium. Special packs by order of the Doctor.

X. DEGENERATION OF THE GELATIGENOUS TISSUE.

Another group of organ's of vast importance is the one which consists of gelatigenous tissue. In fact all blood and lymphatic vessels, air alveoli of the lungs, tendons and cords of the whole system, the digestive tract from the mouth to the anus, the stomach, the bladder, and indeed every organ or tissue which has the function of expansion and contraction, must be made of gelatigenous (rubber-like) tissue. Otherwise it cannot perform its duties in the organism and must needs become degenerate.

While there are not many special forms of disease of the gelatigenous tissue itself, many diseased conditions occur in connection with its degeneration. This in turn is caused by the lack of gelatigenous food, which the blood must convey to this tissue wherever it exists in the body.

It is obvious that any degeneration which may affect the intestinal duct, the bladder or other organs which contain gelatine in their composition will require gelatigenous regeneration.

The principal forms of disease which may affect the organs in question are those which have been discussed under catarrhal diseases (Section VI). The acute and chronic forms of stomach and intestinal disease, especially, belong to this group, and have consequently received special attention. The treatment of this question in my work, "Regeneration" or "Dare To Be Healthy," Chapter X, A and B, will answer, in detail the questions of those who desire more enlightenment on this most vital and intricate subject.

Therapy.

Diet: These forms include all catarrhal disease mentioned under VI. A, also all inflammatory conditions of the stomach and intestines, in their acute form. As far as the latter are concerned, the suitable lists of diet will be found under Forms II, III, IV, V and VI. Regarding the same diseases in the chronic form, the special diet lists are given under Forms IV, V and VI. In addition the following suggestions will be helpful:

Diseases of the Stomach and Intestines.

These prescriptions of diet serve especially for the diseases of the stomach and intestines. In most cases a prescription for the rational preparation of food is such as only the hygienic physician is able to give. Food for persons suffering from diseases of the stomach, must be selected individually according to their idiosyncrasies. In one case the stomach must be prevented from doing too much; in another case it must be stimulated. In one case the object is to fatten; in another, to remove fat. In some cases the physician prescribes food which will retard the movement of the bowels, in other instances, the patient requires food that will promote such movement. The diet for patients with fever must be different from the diet for convalescing patients. People suffering from diabetes require a peculiar preparation of their food. Not everything that is good for an adult will be beneficial to a child. The digestibility of many foods depends upon their preparation. The value of food for patients can be judged rightly from but one standpoint, that of digestibility.

The fundamental principles governing the nourishment for patients are digestibility, great variety, abolition of all strong spices, nutritive and well selected material.

The temperature of drinks must be in strict accordance with the prescription of the physician. The patient must be urged to thoroughly masticate the food, so that it will be properly salivated and thus facilitate digestion. Patients seriously ill, should receive their food mashed or minced, so that they can partake of it more easily. All waste parts, such as skin, fat, sinews, bones, must be removed from the food, even for convalescents. Warmed up food and fibrous vegetables must be banished from the patient's diet. It must not be a question as to what the patient wants; the prescription of the physician only must govern. The patient's food must be prepared carefully, absolutely correctly and in a cleanly manner. In case of strong thirst, great care must be exercised in regard to drinks, depending on the physician's directions. The thirsty feeling of the patient may be alleviated by putting glyzerine on his lips and small pieces of ice on his tongue, without, however, permitting him to swallow the water as the ice melts.

Normal Diet for Stomach Diseases.

Milk, sweet and sour, buttermilk, yoghurt, kefir, albumen cacao, cereals in the form of mush, strained legumes, cooked in soup or milk, all sorts of glutinous soups, farinose dishes prepared from stale rolls, biscuits, zwieback, tender and easily, digestible meats, mashed game meat, chicken, raw beef, ham, meat jelly, young vegetables, preserved fruit.

Avoid the following: all indigestible fats, meat which requires more than 4 to 5 hours for its digestion, hot salads, gas-producing vegetables, gravy, fruits which abound in cellulose, such as apricots and peaches, hard stems, xylocarp ribs of leaves, the strong smelling and sharp tasting parts of some kinds of vegetables, as for instance, new potatoes, cabbage (in the cooking of which the first water must be poured off), hot soups and spicy herbs, spices of all kinds, high game, sausages, bacon, yeast pastry, drinks too hot or too cold, strong coffee (in the place of which fruit coffee is recommended), stale raisins and almonds, nuts, too much candy, much liquid with meats, and excitement of all kinds while eating.

General Hints for a nourishing treatment.

The patient who is to gain in flesh must adhere strictly to the prescribed diet as well as to the prescribed rest, if the treatment is to take effect.

The following articles are very nourishing: yolks of eggs prepared in any style, milk, cream, kefir, rich cheese, beef marrow on toast (cooked in soup), all kinds of noodles and dumplings, puddings, cocoa and chocolate, white bread, rich thick soups, gravy, potatoes and oats prepared in various ways, sweet beer, malt beer, sweet wines and puddings with preserved fruits, fruit juices, meat from well-fed animals only. All meals must be served in small portions, so as not to create distaste for food.

7 *A.M.* — 250 grams of fresh, boiled, unskimmed milk, or ¼ quart cocoa prepared with milk or Knorr's oat-cocoa, or ⅛ quart cream with tea added, one roll, butter and honey.

9 *A.M.* — 1 cup bouillon, 20 grams hot or cold roast meat, 30 grams Graham or gluten bread, 10 grams butter. Then ¼ quart milk, butter and Graham bread.

11 *A.M.* — ¼ quart milk with the yolk of one egg.

1 *P.M.* — 100 grams soup (oat, barley, vegetable soup), green corn, sago soup, 100 grams potatoes, 100 grams tender vegetables, such as spinach, mashed peas, mashed carrots, mashed artichokes, asparagus tips strained, 20 grams easily digestable rice, 50 grams preserved fruit; or, no soup, but, instead meat, vegetables, apple sauce, dishes made from milk or flour, such as noodles, fruit, ⅛ quart cream.

4 *P.M.* — Light tea or milk, with malt or cocoa added, two crackers, ½ quart milk.

6 *P.M.* — 20 grams meat (hot or cold roast meat), raw meat or 10 grams Graham bread, 10 grams butter, milk chocolate, Graham bread, butter, honey.

8 *P.M.* — 1 cup soup with 10 grams butter and one yolk, barley, oats, etc., eggs or meat, vegetables, preserved fruits, Graham bread, butter, mild cream cheese.

9.30 *P.M.* — ¼ quart milk, with a spoonful of malt extract, ⅛ quart cream.

As a special breakfast, for a thin patient, the following drink is recommended: To a cup of unskimmed hot milk add one yolk and one spoonful of pure bee-honey. This must be taken in the morning on an empty stomach for several weeks.

In case of Constipation.

If constipation is due to nervousness or sluggishness of the bowels, the best means to overcome the trouble is mixed coarse food, using various mineral waters, and little meat, but plenty of vegetables, especially sauerkraut, cabbage, comfrey, cauliflower, pumpkin, tomatoes, cucumbers, various salads and fruits, jellies. Among beverages sour milk, buttermilk, kefir No. I and II, yoghurt, various new wines, fruit juices, different mineral waters, such as Apollinaris, Karlsbad waters, Hunyady; coarse bread, such as Graham, avoiding fine white bread. In extremely chronic cases use my Laxagen Tea in case of emergency.

Dech-Manna-Compositions: **Gelatinogen**, **Plasmogen**, Mucogen, Eubiogen.

Physical: Abdominal packs, with vinegar and water.

Acute — warm.

Chronic — cold.

XI. DEGENERATION OF THE CARTILAGINOUS TISSUE.

Cartilage in the human body is the material which must cover the end of each bone so as to prevent its destruction by friction. It is the important part in all joints. It is obvious that any degeneration of this particular tissue will cause friction, which is combined with severe pains, called Ankylosis, Gout.

The degeneration is usually a consequence of improper proportion of the various food ingredients consumed, omitting the material necessary for the construction of the cartilage, which, being in use, is constantly used up rapidly. Regeneration of the blood, by assisting it in its important task of feeding the cartilaginous tissues, and regulation of the diet are the only two possible remedies for this form of disease, of such frequent occurrence, the alleged cure for which attracts thousands to bathing resorts, where they derive not the slightest real benefit.

The variety of gout called arthritis (deforming gout), is the most pronounced and dangerous phase of this form of disease.

Therapy.

Diet: The diet is exactly the same as prescribed for rheumatism and gout under V, Degeneration of the Muscular Tissue.

Dech-Manna-Compositions: **Cartilogen**, **Plasmogen**, Gelatinogen, Eubiogen.

Physical: Partial packs, salt and radium, massage, oxygenator bath, half bath radium and salt.

In case of arthritis, also special packs according to the directions of the Doctor. It is impossible to give a diet for arthritic patients, peculiarities of this disease being largely individual.

XII. DEGENERATION OF THE BODY TISSUE IN GENERAL.

By "body tissue in general" is understood the body with the total sum of its cells—especially the red blood corpuscles—and their various aggregations. Consequently a special composition of nutritive salts, under the name of Eubiogen, has been composed, which is the most perfect duplication of all the chemical elements of the entire body in the correct proportion. Eubiogen, therefore, is prescribed as a secondary Dech-Manna-Composition, to be taken with all other compositions. But it also acts independently as the best means of preventing degeneration, and in this capacity should not be missing in the diet of adults as well as of children. The cost thus incurred would be recouped many times over through its prevention of disease.

Eubiogen takes a leading position in reference to the following complicated forms of disease, in the treatment of which it becomes the most important factor among the nutritive compositions: Ataxia, Basedow's Disease, Diabetes Mellitus, Obesity, Bright's Disease, Arterio-Sclerosis. I am prepared to explain to patients, this curative method and the reasons for its application; but these complicated diseases, while based on the same degenerations of blood, and consequently of the tissue and organs, as all others, offer impressions which, from the point of view of the conscientious physician, cannot be presented with but a few bare words of explanation. Nor does the space at my disposal permit me to go into the matter with due thoroughness.

All of these ailments have been described in my work: "Regeneration or Dare To Be Healthy."

The intelligent reader will readily conceive that he who has found the secret of the degenerations constituting the various forms of disease, will not hesitate before their complications. *Ataxia, Basedow's Disease, Diabetes Mellitus, Obesity, Bright's Disease and Arterio-Sclerosis, can be cured. They can be cured by the same methods of which simpler examples have been already given.*

No one, who in the struggle for health has surrendered to the attack of constitutional disease, the germ of which may have been implanted in him by his forefathers, needs despair. Let him seek advice before too late, and the strong probability is that in due time he will have regained his health, and will be enabled to fulfil his duties to himself and to posterity.

NOTE. — In reference to the foregoing tables of dietary "Regimen" the reader must clearly understand that the prescriptions are merely indications of diet appropriate to various phases of the complaints to the treatment of which they are attached; but the decision as to how and when these phases occur in individual cases should be left entirely to the discretion of the physician in charge of the case who will, of course, also pronounce upon the diet. Should there be no such authority present, the greatest care and common sense must be devoted to the selection from the said tables of a system of diet suitable to the various stages of disease. Any recommendations therein contained which may appear to be contradictory or conflicting must be ascribed to their complication on a progressive dietary system consistent with the prospective advancement of the case towards recovery.

INFANTILE PARALYSIS.

Amongst the forms of Degeneration of the Muscular Tissue the reader will have noticed that of Infantile Paralysis or Poliomyelitis.

The startling prominence that this complaint quite recently acquired was due to its world-wide ravages in epidemic form and the absolute and confessed inability of the combined sagacity of the whole faculty of the orthodox medical profession to cope with it or to cure it—to fathom its cause and origin or to curtail its increasing rate of mortality. I am therefore constrained, so far as space permits, to give the matter special and particular consideration.

The scientific name, "Poliomyelitis," is derived from the Greek words: polios, grey and myleos, marrow; for its chief feature is a softening of the grey spinal marrow.

First noticed by the medical world no later than the year 1840, statistics show that in the last decade it has appeared in various parts of the world in epidemic form, notably in Sweden and Norway. In America, epidemics occurred in 1907 and 1908 and again in 1916. It was promptly and energetically dealt with by the Rockefeller Institute of New York where the proof was established of the possibility of transmission by a living virus taken from the spinal marrow of a victim; but whether this disseminator may be correctly termed a bacillus, or fungus or a germ, medical-science has been unable lo determine; neither has it succeeded with the most powerful microscope in discovering the individuality of this "carrier," whilst all experiments with re-agents have been bare of results. Thus the researches of science have merely brought us back to the starting point; namely, that there is a "something" which exerts a degenerating influence upon the cellular tissue of the spinal marrow and causes the morbid enlargement of its cells.

The New York Board of Health, cites eight different forms in which the disease may appear and acknowledges a startling failure to determine either any uniform period of incubation (i.e. the time between contagion and the appearance of the symptoms,) or the period of infection (i.e. how long a sick person may be a danger to others).

The New York press accepts the situation philosophically; as follows:

"Infantile Paralysis cannot be cured by means of medicines. The physician must of necessity limit his ministrations to easing the pain, providing for easy movement of the bowels and so forth, but otherwise *he must let nature take its course*."

Medical reference books vaguely define the disease with diverse and indefinite theories, showing that science on the subject is practically mute.

But the medically "unprofessional," random remark of the New York press-man has exactly hit the mark: "Let nature take its course."

The fact is that nothing very clear or absolute can be said about Infantile Paralysis; for observation shows that it is apparently a matter of racial conditions and environment and that only from the general application of the Laws of Nature, as taught by biology can we reasonably hope to solve the problem or cure the disease.

As the result of careful study of many cases I simply confirmed the fact that Infantile Paralysis belongs strictly to the class in which in the foregoing chapter I have placed it, and is subject to the same rules, influences and treatment. In most of the cases treated I have not failed to discover the existence of spinal trouble in one or other of the parents. This, engendering *predisposition* to similar complaints *in the children of the opposite sex*, which, acted upon by the irritants bred of poor or irrational nutriment and unhygienic environment in greater or lesser degree, results in attacks of this disease, in plain or epidemic form as the case may be, to which all children so predisposed are liable. Thus, incidentally, is my recently discovered "Law of the Cross-Transmission of Characteristics" amply verified.

As to the cause which leads to the development of this predisposition in the children, the answer, of course, is improper nourishment; and amongst the contributory causes I would specially indicate, "Pasteurized" and "sterilized" milk which has been absolutely banned by science on the basis of Physical Chemistry, according to which it was definitely proved in a report laid before the Paris Academy of Sciences, that valuable bone-forming ingredients in the milk, (a combination of carbonic and phosphoric lime,) are lost in course of Pasteurization, since at the temperature necessary for the process they are *transmuted by heat into insoluble elements*, (phosphate and carbonate of lime) which, precipitated by chemical action, either drop to the bottom in sediment or cling to the surface coating and, in either case, are eliminated and lost to the child to an extent which constitutes a serious deterioration in its food and one likely in any case to promote rickets. Milk also contains important constituents which change into necessary food elements in the course of natural fermentation—gelatine for instance—which being, as has been shown, so vital a factor in the building up of tissue, it needs no argument to prove the disastrous consequences its depletion must engender in the child and it may be likewise safely left to the intelligence of the reader to grasp the obvious fact that for the prevention or healing of Infantile Paralysis the one and only safeguard is Regeneration through the course already indicated of Hygienic-Dietetic treatment which will, if applied beforehand, eliminate the tendency to disease or, in the event of its occurrence, will conduct it along safe and natural lines to a quick recovery.

This brief sketch of the subject must suffice for the present purpose but a special article [C] with full and interesting details has been devoted to the subject, which will appear in my greater work, "Regeneration or Dare to be Healthy."

"FACIAL DIAGNOSIS" AND "THE CLINICAL EYE."

It is an incident common to the experience of all Natural Hygienic Physicians for the patient to exclaim in quasi protest: "But Doctor! How can you tell?"

Accustomed to the pompous pantomime of the orthodox physician—the gold watch and chain trick, while pulse and tongue reveal their hidden records—and then the well known questions which call forth the personal predilection in the fashion of disease and diet, (prescriptions which are often not untinged by the physician's own proclivities), at first the patient misses the old familiar presence. If ill he *must* be, he expects that the process should proceed from the outset on the old accustomed, "strictly respectable" lines, and something like resentment stirs him when, in place of questioning, a physician presumes to *tell him* at a glance the substance of his malady *unasked*.

But such is the method of real efficiency and such the qualification of the men who practice the new philosophy which shall save the world from shams.

Facial diagnosis is the determining factor of the logical and never failing science of natural therapy which is coming to the rescue of mankind, in spite of legal and commercial obstruction.

The "Clinical Eye" is, emphatically, *not* the sad old "Eye of Faith" which has sent its millions to their doom, but the *sober, steady, practiced introspective hopeful eye of knowledge and experience*.

The external symptoms visible to the clinical eye of a physician worthy of the name, vastly outweigh in important significance, all the objectionable detailed examination of parts and organs which from long use has become the habit of the old-school practitioner. Moreover the swift impressions gathered under the clinical eye are spontaneous and reliable whereas, as the result of questioning or the description of the patient, they possibly are not, but rather represent too often some preconceived notion of alleged heredity or devotional pessimism, sometimes original but more probably the suggestion of relatives and friends.

The subject is a vitally important one and, with a view to clearing away the obstruction of old superstitions from the mind of the reader, I shall trespass upon my allotted space in order to give a brief extract of my remarks thereon as expressed in my greater work: "Regeneration or Dare to be Healthy."

DIAGNOSIS, PHYSIOGNOMY AND PSYCHOLOGY.

The biological healing system, based on the laws of nature and the acknowledgment of the fact that no two cases of disease are exactly alike, requires much broader knowledge and much deeper insight on the part of the physician than did the old-school of medicine with its search for symptoms of special diseases and its occult prescriptions.

Since the object is to get at the root of the evil in order to regenerate the patient thoroughly, it becomes imperative to obtain, what is hardest to elicit from him perhaps, the accurate truth about himself and his ailment.

And though expert in recognizing external symptoms, it is unwise to rely entirely thereon and research must continue into realms where the patient himself only can lead us and where, willing or otherwise, he is apt to mislead.

Psychology teaches how to find the way into the darkness of a patient's soul. Physiognomy teaches, not only to read in the face and external appearance, the story of a life which is written there in characters which only experience may decipher, but also to realize when the patient employs physiognomical expressions to hide what we persistently seek; namely, the truth.

And again, in regard to healing, psychology teaches how to influence the patient so that he may discontinue to be his own worst enemy; that he may recognize his mistakes as such and discard them, although possibly he may have grown so addicted to his tastes as to prefer to continue therein in place of daring to be healthy.

In the plan of production of a regenerated and healthy humanity, every individual of this kind must be regarded as a foe who interferes with the prevention of disease both now and in futurity. To win such an one over, to make him an enthusiastic believer in the theory that health is a necessity, and, a task less easy, to prevent his relapse into his previous degenerate manner of life and health,—

this is another branch of science for which psychology and physiognomy are more needful than anything else.

Here again it is the true physician's principle to enlighten the layman, and not to surround his methods with a mysterious, but imposing wall of secrecy.

We do not hesitate to reveal the main points of our system of diagnosis, which is much broader than the old system of scholastic medicine, — the performance with auscultation, percussion, X rays and the rest. Certain knowledge of these things will lead every one, ere long, to submit all disturbances of health to the hygienic physician while prevention is still probable and possible, instead of waiting until disease has taken firm hold. It will also enable men to realize that the old-school practitioner who pronounces them sound while they feel for themselves that there is something wrong within has yet "a something" left to learn.

The realm of psychology, however, is beyond the scope of my present endeavour, save in so far as it may serve to show that we are fortified with this particular knowledge, and to the end that this book may constitute a help to the aspiring hygienic-dietetic physician, calling his attention to the necessity of acquiring as profound a knowledge of psychology as may be.

I will confine myself at present, therefore, to the external symptoms which must be observed, though they are not generally considered as symptoms of disease; and yet they indicate disease or the disposition thereto, individual or hereditary, as the case may be.

I shall consequently deal with the peculiarities of hands and feet, nails and hair, eyes and ears, nose and teeth, mouth, forehead, tongue, chin, cheeks, neck, chest, abdomen, legs, and general constitution.

Nature has endowed us with strong discriminating faculties against certain external indications of disease. We experience a pleasant feeling when the hand is pressed by another hand that is warm and dry, but we shrink from the hand that is cold and moist and clammy.

Perspiring hands and feet are a sure indication that some process of degeneration is going on within the body, the production of diseased cells being in excess of what the body, under normal conditions, is able to excrete, and therefore they seek unusual channels of leaving the body, that is, through the skin and mucous membranes.

Perspiring feet are a symptom of disposition to colds and possibly tuberculosis, while perspiring hands indicate certain nervous diseases and disposition to gout; constantly cold hands and feet are usually found in people who suffer from scrofulosis or anaemia.

In many cases the quality of *nails* leads to the conclusion that there is a thorough disturbance of the process of nutrition. If they are fragile and brittle, there is no question but that there is lack of certain nutritive salts in the blood. Swollen and deformed nails indicate special disturbances in circulation, chronic heart and lung diseases.

Hair, or rather the absence of hair, especially in early life, is sometimes another indication of faulty nutrition.

Baldness or premature gray hair is usually a pathological indication, as is also the dishevelled hair of nervous people and children suffering from scrofulosis, while rich, glossy hair is always a sign of good health.

The development of the hair depends upon the activity of the skin, the nerves and the composition of the blood. The blood of dark-haired people is lacking in water and fat, but richer in albuminous matter. Poor quality of hair is indicative of living in bad air, poor nutrition of the skin, hard mental work, pain and sorrow. Sexual excesses during youth are often the cause of premature baldness and thin hair.

The *eyes* present a picture that manifests the general condition of the body, whether it be healthy, disposed to disease, or suffering from disease.

Protruding eyes are the sure symptom of the disease known as Basedow's disease; they indicate also short-sightedness, and hereditary epilepsy.

The condition of the mucous membranes of the eyes permits certain conclusions as to the genital organs.

If the eyes are abnormally small, we draw the conclusion that there is general weakness and deficiency in nutrition. They indicate retarded development, which may be seated in the central nervous system. The eyes usually recede during severe diseases. A hyperaemic condition of the eyelids, with or without inflammation, is always a symptom of a dysaemic condition of the entire system (scrofulosis). In some cases of scrofulosis there is not another visible sign on the entire body, and yet the eyelids and eyelashes, which sticks together most of the time, tell the story of an inherited condition of dysaemia.

A yellowish hue of the eyes indicates disease of the liver.

The color of the iris does not indicate much in itself, although the theory of Liljequist, which deserves some attention, claims that if a person deteriorates in health, the eyes, if originally light blue, darken more and more and finally change into brown or the color of the hybrid race. Liljequist's scale of healthy eyes reads: Light blue, medium blue, dark blue; then light, medium and dark brown. However, brown eyes do not represent sickness; they but indicate nervousness and sensibility.

According to Liljequist, individuals belong to the hybrid race when they are born of parents one of whom has blue eyes and the other brown eyes. The weaker race transmits the brown colour of its iris to the middle part of the iris of the child, while the colour of the stronger race reappears in the outer part of the iris; not, however, as pure blue, but tinted with a delicate shade of green, in consequence of the light brownish-yellowish colour which emanates from the central part.

When death is imminent, the iris displays a grayish-black, muddy gray or muddy brown colour.

The pupil of the eye is irritated in cases of nervous disease and indicates this condition. In cases where only one pupil is dilated, a local disease of the optic nerve or one side of the brain is evident. If the pupils are insensible to external irritations and remain rigid, the conclusion is that the brain or the spinal cord is badly affected.

It may be stated in a general way that clear, brilliant eyes, (when not caused by fever) are usually an indication of the good quality of the blood as well as of all other humours of the body, together with normal activity of all the central organs.

The *mouth* and *tongue*: Pathological indications manifested by the mouth are principally displayed by the lips, which are clear red in healthy people, while a hectic red indicates fever and pulmonary disease. Pale lips indicate anaemia and chlorosis, and lips of a bluish hue are signs of a generally weakened organism. Frequent, vivid contractions of the lips (usually thin in this case) indicate great nervousness.

The color of the mucous membrane of the tongue is a very fair indication of health or sickness. If a person is in health, the tongue is rosy and not coated. But any disturbance in the intestines causes a more or less coated tongue, and consequently shows the detrimental influence these particular ailments exert upon the brain and nerves. Hence, a coated tongue affords a valuable indication in making a correct diagnosis, especially in case of chronic catarrh of the stomach, this being one of the main causes of depression, and melancholia, as stated by Piderit.

The *forehead*, or rather the record traced thereon, in lines of nature's unimpeachable calligraphy, warrants certain conclusions as to mentality and character; and these may be important in determining the truthfulness of the patient's stories of suffering and other items which facilitate or impede a correct diagnosis.

The interpretation of such features, however, belongs to the realm of pure psychology, this is also true of similar conclusions drawn from the outlines of the chin.

Of much more importance for the purpose of diagnosis is the *nose*.

Even a child understands what the red nose of the habitual drunkard signifies. A bloated nose with a tendency to become sore is an indication of a disposition to scrofulosis.

Other indications of disease are displayed to the experienced physician by the condition of the nose.

The *nose* is one of the most typical of the human organs; it is also in the closest connection with the entire system with its groups of organs — the brain, intestines, breast and even the sexual organs.

The infinite variety of nasal formation has attracted the intense interest of the physiognomist to this organ.

The most important function of the nose lies in its action as a respiratory organ. Bad habits or faulty construction which prevent it from serving in this capacity, lead to much suffering and disease, and it is always important to determine whether the channels of the nose are clear and open and efficiently serve their purposes.

The function of the nose as an olfactory organ must also rank highly in its importance. In this case, however, the nose of the physician plays the important part; not the nose of the patient. In fact, most of the famous authorities, among them Professor Jaeger of Stuttgart, Dr. Heim of Berlin and Dr. Lahmann of Dresden, have made very valuable discoveries in this respect.

Dr. Heim has found methods of determining the nature of certain acute diseases from the odour emitted from the person.

Dr. Lahmann distinguishes the hypochondriacal, the melancholic and the hysteric odours, which, as he says, are most characteristic.

The same applies to the odour of diabetics and other people who suffer from disturbances of digestion, and patients who suffer from cancer and other diseases involving a process of putrefaction.

The fact that most patients diffuse unpleasant odours is of the greatest importance to married people, as it easily produces antipathy, and especially in the case of chronic diseases, is frequently made the basis of separation and divorce.

Were this defect known to be but the symptom of a curable disease, the husband or wife would probably prefer to consult the hygienic physician rather than the lawyer. Knowledge in such case would mean the preservation of domestic happiness.

The teeth: The parents of a young man once complained to me that their son had been rejected as a cadet at West Point upon physical examination, because two of his teeth were filled.

The authorities are certainly justified in their decision.

The lack of perfect teeth indicates faulty digestion. Usually the teeth are ruined during youth because children breathe through the mouth instead of through the nose, — either on account of the physical condition of the nose or because the tonsils are enlarged.

The lack of sufficient nutritive salts in the diet is often revealed by the condition of the teeth.

From a physiological standpoint the teeth are no less important than the brain, the eyes and the hair; and the conclusion that perfect eyes, hair and teeth indicate a perfect brain is absolutely justified, while the lack of perfection in these organs shows internal deficiencies long before they appear in external manifestation in the form of disease.

Since healthy blood is the basic condition of healthy teeth, the fact that people have clean white teeth, set in regular line, indicates the existence of healthy blood. On the other hand, a bad composition of the blood is manifested by short, irregularly set, yellowish teeth.

The teeth of healthy people are always somewhat moist, dry teeth are accordingly a bad sign.

The only advantage of yellowish teeth rests in the fact that their dentine is, as a rule, stronger. Extremely bluish white teeth often consist of a soft, porous and tender dentine.

Faulty structure of the teeth indicates weak bones in general.

Crippled teeth and the late appearance of teeth in infants, — that is, not before the ninth month, — are symptoms of rachitis. Healthy children have their teeth between the fifth and seventh months.

The teeth of diabetics become loose without any formation of tartar, (an incrustation of phosphate of lime and saliva).

Extremely yellow teeth indicate jaundice, while reddish teeth show hyperaemia of the dentine. Carious teeth are a result of disturbed circulation.

The gums are also very indicative of disease. If they are of a pale pink colour, they indicate anaemia or chlorosis; if bluish red on the edge, they indicate tuberculosis.

Some of the most striking indications of existing disease are demonstrated by the *neck*. By feeling the neck and carefully watching its external appearance, the experienced scientist will obtain much valuable information that will aid in his diagnosis, and give him additional knowledge as to the processes going on within the body of the patient.

The significance of the formation of the *thorax* (*chest*) is well known, even to many laymen. Flat chest, so-called chicken chest, indicates imperfect development of the lungs, and when extreme, even tuberculosis.

A flabby abdomen indicates disposition to hernia and stagnation of the blood, frequently causing hemorrhoids or inflammation of the prostate gland in men, and all kinds of diseases — inflammatory or catarrhal — in women.

As to the *legs*, the so-called varicose veins are indications of weak blood-vessels and intestinal hemorrhage, while inflamed nerves lead to the conclusion of gouty diathesis and the danger of paralytic strokes.

The *skin* usually affords more indications that aid in forming a correct diagnosis than is usually recognized.

If examination were made of the excreta through the pores of an individual during 24 hours, some conclusion might be definitely arrived at as to any germs of disease present in the body and in course of expulsion in this way.

All bacteria incident to detrimental processes proceeding within the human organism, are to be found in the perspiration.

Freckles indicate a certain predisposition inherent in the blood, while some forms of eczema point to the conclusion that there are diseased processes in action within the body.

It is most important under this system to determine the chemical condition of the body in each individual case.

Acids or alkalines prevail. If the former, patients have bad teeth, a disposition to gout, diabetes and cancer. The normal condition is the predominance of alkalines.

In such cases as the former, physiological chemistry will point to the counterbalancing of the acids to establish a correct composition of the blood, and thus to prevent the impending danger. The biological system of health which is rapidly taking the place of all others, is equipped with so searching a knowledge of the human organism that no disease, be it ever so adroitly concealed, can escape its minute attention; not excepting even the disposition to disease.

The old adage is still true that "prevention is better than cure" and the intelligent person will probably recognize the wisdom of so safe and sane a course and endeavor to prevent the evils to which he may be exposed. Thus, for his own satisfaction, if he be wise he will adopt these two simple precautions:

(1) Examination by an accredited hygienic-dietetic physician.

(2) Regulation of his mode of living in accordance with the course prescribed.

The words of the famous Moleschott ring true today, more than in the past, when he said: "One of the principal questions a patient should ask his physician is, how to make good, healthy blood." Experience shows that there is but one method to attain good blood, — that *priceless factor* upon which our *thinking*, our *feeling*, our *power* and our *progeny depend*, and that is by means of *correct food and nutrition*.

FOOTNOTES:

[B] See special article on Influenza, page 408.

[C] This article is also printed in pamphlet form and may be had from the author for 50c. Postage paid.

CHILDREN'S DISEASE.

"The cause of the Poor to plead on,
'twixt Deity and Demon."

(Carlyle).

"Child of mortality whence contest thou,
Why is thy countenance sad, and why are
Thine eyes red with weeping?"

(Bartauld).

I have opened this chapter with somewhat startling mottos, for its pathetic theme is Children and children's disease; and it seems to me appropriate, in view of what it portends, to send forth in this form a world-thought, as a harbinger of sympathy—a foreword which may set in motion the thought-waves of pity. For of all living creatures born into this world of pompous ignorance and maudlin solicitude to struggle for precarious existence from the cradle to the grave, by reason of the unnatural conditions of our vaunted hygienic and educational systems—generously termed "civilization"—there is surely nothing quite so "poor," so woefully devoid of practical protection, and, in its exceptional helplessness, so weakly gushed over and little understood as the child of frail humanity.

"The cause of the poor"—thus the legend runs—"in deity's or demon's name." For truly, of the two angels which, we are told, attend upon the birth of credulous mankind and the initial stages of development, the malign influence would seem to be ever in the ascendant, irrespective of the social status of the, more or less, prenatally affected, innocent reproduction wherein is focused the latent follies and delinquencies of the race, as portrayed in the course of its long pangenesis.

Now, incredible though it may seem and deplorable though it be, the secret which has revealed itself with absolute force and conviction to the judicial minds of unemotional scientific observers is simply this: that the children of the present generation are, as an incontestable matter of actual fact, really brought into this world alive and some attain to maturity, not through maternal intelligence, but rather, *in spite of mothers.* This is a hard saying but none the less a truth. They survive in spite of the idiosyncracies of their fondly irrational, untutored mothers rather than because of any practical, efficient effort these contribute towards the well being and survival of their offspring. This, as a general rule, is unhappily beyond question. It is a rule which has, naturally, many exceptions, — many brave and brilliant ones — these however only serve to confirm it.

Comte, writing as an authority on the subject, made the assertion that there is hardly an example on record of a child of superior genius whose mother did not possess also a superior order of mind. As an example he cites: The mother of Napoleon Bonaparte, high-souled, heroic and beautiful; the mother of Julius Caesar, a singularly fine character, wise and strong; the mother of Goethe, — affectionately termed: "The delight of her children, the favourite of poets and princes — one whose splendid talents and characteristics were reproduced in her son." There are also, we know full well, unnumbered hosts of others, whose kindly light has been shed in many an humble or secluded home, whose beloved names have been called blessed by thousands though unrecorded in historic page — who have lived and loved and passed on to higher realms — to the world, to eulogy and to fame unknown.

In ancient days, when Athens was the centre of culture and of learning, the Greek mothers were more prone to regard the significance of pre-natal influences than are the mothers of the present day of putative advancement. The hereditary tendencies of child-life, with all its complexities of racial and ancestral character and the qualities resulting from the dual source of parentage, were then perhaps better understood, or at least more seriously considered; also the obvious but grossly disregarded fact that the cradled infant of today may be the responsible citizen of the future, was kept more effectively in mind and its significance to the State more fully recognized. The wisdom of Solomon was never more clearly demonstrated than when he said: "Train up a child in the way he should go; and when he is old, he will not depart from it." It is a piece of world philosophy which has reigned unquestioned throughout the ages—a policy upon which human discernment, in Church and State, has relied with unfailing effect; "for the thoughts of a child are long, long thoughts"—those well-remembered words, how true; for those "long thoughts"—the mental environment of the formative period of child-life—do inevitably determine the future character of the individual, and the immediate result of neglect in these vitally important stages is painfully and promptly apparent in the aggressive and unchildlike deportment of the turbulent young neophytes of both sexes, so disproportionately in evidence in all directions throughout the community of the present, as to bring into ridicule and utter contempt existing methods of control. This dire defect in individual restraint may be largely ascribed to both physical and mental degeneracy, of hereditary origin; and when to this is added the attempts of parents to maintain the tranquility of the home by threats, bribery and fatuous promises—undue severity on the one hand and undue licence on the other—serious developments are not far to seek. It has been well said that children who are governed through their appetites in their infancy are usually governed by their appetites in maturity. Thus it is, by unwise methods of control which appeal wholly to the spirit of greed, emulation and selfishness in the child—the purely animal instincts—with perhaps the occasional degrading influence of corporal punishment, as a later development, that so many young lives are wrecked and the downward path made easy which leads through duplicity to crime. The infantile precosity of the age leaves little scope for the old-time sentimental prudery of parents who fail to discriminate between innocence and ignorance; but it has been stated by a well known American authority on the subject of child-culture, whose experience of child-life and schools is nation-wide, that only about one child in a hundred receives proper instruction early enough to protect it from vice. Then again there supervenes the evil of the competitive school system which, too frequently, forces the education of a child beyond the natural order of growth. Countless numbers of little ones are injured by enforced premature development, thereby diverting the vital forces to the development of the brain which should be devoted to the development of the body.

Encompassed by such a chain of adverse circumstances as the combined result of parental egotism and pedantic, pedagogical ignorance, is it wonderful, I would ask, that the ghastly record of the hideous sacrifice of child-life is what it is, and that the young lives which do by chance escape the horrible holocaust, still reap the prevailing harvest of prolific ills of which the coming explanation will give some adequate conception.

Often the fondly futile questions fall from the anxious lips of maternal foreboding: What has the future in store for me? Will my child live? Will providence grant me this long-sought blessing? A thousand such thoughts continually assail the heart in a mother's intense solicitude; but not in vain will her hopes be set, if haply, she may reverently follow the course of Mother Nature's laws and precepts, into which I will endeavor to give you some insight.

Every thinking man must shudder to find it recorded in statistical tables how insane asylums and prisons are overflowing, how suicides and crimes against life and soul are but common incidents. It is not hard for each one of us to see the demon of greed and avarice in the eyes of those we meet, ready and eager to snatch away the very bread from the lips of his fellow man because he, too, is hungry and lacking life's necessities. The egotism of mankind grows constantly stronger; all are in haste to become rich, that thus they may enjoy life before its little span is spent. What has become of the youths exuberant in strength, who once were wont to set out, all jubilant with song, in their heyday of freedom, to revel in nature and bathe their lungs in its balsamic atmosphere—to return strengthened to their sleep at early evening, and who really sought to retain their health? They who were the pride of their parents, the joy of their sisters, the blissful hope of a waiting bride. Can we recognize such in the average youth of today,—the citizen of the tomorrow—these effigies of men, degraded by the demons of alcohol and nicotine, by the gambling passion, and by the company of loose women, into dissipated dissolute invalids unwholesome in themselves and a menace to the race?

Let us pass on rather to the gentler sex.

Where are the sprightly, modest maidens with cheeks rosy with healthy blood, graceful in figure with well developed forms—the chaste, pure spirit shining in their eyes, with witchery and common sense combined? Where are the fathers and mothers whose good fortune it is to possess such children as these? Can it be that they should deem these caricatures of fashion worthy of their fond desire? — these whose days are spent in idling, who find their pleasure in the streets, the shops, the theatres and the like they term "society?"

Those men are old at forty years.

Those youths too often die at twenty, dissipated wrecks, holding as a mere ceremony the marriage they expect eventually to consummate; or married, now and then produce a single child that had far better never have been born.

What of those mothers who cannot nourish their own offspring, but fain would make shift with all imaginable unnatural substitutes and bring up children in whom a predisposition to disease has already been born?

Oh nature! High and mighty mistress! A bitter penalty dost thou exact from these thine erring progeny.

And rightly so.

Cruelly plain dost thou stamp thy mark on the tiny brow of the unborn child to mark in what degree its parents have departed from thine eternal ways of truth.

When a great man, recently, in his address before the body of a famous university, solemnly asserted that mankind is growing better, day by day, he must have had before his inner eye fair visions of a future race — the Future of Truth, which come it must — some day — but now lies dormant in the lap of the gods, its alluring, visionary, transcendental form depicted, for an optimistic instant, in the fervent, hopeful heart of a sincere but far-sighted reformer. But it is written: false prophets must come, deceiving in respect to all things in heaven and earth. "Mundus vult decipi, ergo decipiatur." (The world wishes to be deceived, therefore, let it be deceived.) The world elects to be deceived. It is so — often on the most paltry of pretences. And here lies the fatal and prolific cause which has ever, throughout the ages, wrought infinite harm and impeded the progress of the world: *The world's indifference to truth.*

For the proper understanding and radical cure of any disease it is of primary importance to have before the mind's eye a distinct picture of its character and developments, thus tracing it back step by step to its source, so that the therapeutic, or healing measures employed may be properly adjusted to its various stages.

Nature has her foes, chief amongst which are ignorance, indulgence and fear; and these foes have ever waged fierce warfare upon her from time immemorial. But today a positive spiritual revolution is being wrought among men, for Mother Nature is calling defaulting humanity back to herself with no uncertain voice.

Back to Nature is now the cry.

Never before were homilies on food so manifold and the ability to profit by them so diminished; never were remedies so abundant and conditions of health so bad; never were deeds of charity so numerous and the poor so discontented; never were measures of reform so prominent and their results so meagre; never was production of commodities so enormous and the cost of living so excessive; never were the resources of all the world so accessible and counterfeits so plentiful; never was enlightenment so widely diffused and sound judgment so restricted; never were the avenues of truth so open, yet never was falsehood so widespread, as in our time.

Our age — well named by Dr. Rudolph Weil, the Age of Nerves — has brought to our service the most significant development of natural forces — electricity in all its forms of application, to medicine and industry and traffic; the expression of motive power in terms of machinery — railroads, ocean travel, air navigation, and endless appliances from the almost limitless scope of which, in the hands of man, the master, not even the very wild beasts escape. Meanwhile however — most strange anomaly — mankind degenerates in body and still more in mind.

The race has become diseased, is suffering, cries out for a betterment of its conditions, grows constantly more embittered and renounces its faith in the powers, human and divine.

Epidemics of terrific proportions sweep their recurring millions into the arms of death; diseases of stupendous mortality, such as tuberculosis, cancer, syphilis, diabetes, and the extensive array of so-called contagious diseases of children, are continually increasing, in spite of doctors, hospitals, sanatoria, hydros, hygienics, asylums, nostrums and serums, and continue to afflict humanity, taking their ghastly toll in daily thousands, despite the vaunted but theoretical advancement of Medical Science.

In the field of medical science the controversy rages at full blast today.

An endless succession of hypotheses, conjectures and dogmas lies widespread before us—a troubled sea of uncertainties—a complex labyrinth of doubt.

The "doctors of medicine" are many but responsible physicians are few, while disease is constantly on the increase among mankind.

It is really little that the people have to learn, for instinct has taught them there is little to be hoped of succour from the professional source. But the world-old habit of superstitious fear and reverence for the "Medicine Man" fetish yet holds its grip upon the race—alike in the savage or the Senate and, despite the knowledge of its fallacy, humanity, still faithful, turns to it weakly, fear-driven, in its hour of distress, knowing no self-reliance and no safer refuge.

The reader will pardon this digression, since it is better that from the outset we should divest ourselves of all delusions and recognize existing conditions as they really are in order that it may help to eliminate these ignorant superstitions from the public mind and implant therein the wholesome fact that there is *no magic in medicine* but simply *an ordinary problem of cause and effect*.

Existence is movement; the whole visible world is progress, development. These are facts which, in truth, are daily becoming more generally known. But man—even modern man—is still so stubbornly unyielding in his faith that what he learns in an instant becomes immovably rooted in his mind to the utter exclusion, generally, of anything new, which even though it be a matter of demonstrated fact, it matters not if at variance with this earlier knowledge; to him it is an impossibility

How often the fallacy of such ultra-conservative principles has been demonstrated has no bearing upon the case; the fact remains— irrational, stupid though it be—that, sublimely indifferent to criticism, it survives, with all the wrong and persecution that follows in its train.

But one of the most noticeable surprises of this description occurred in the year 1896, when Professor Roentgen made public his discovery of the X-rays; for through this discovery facts were disclosed such for instance, as the permeability of solid bodies by luminous rays and the possibility of photographic examination of bony tissues in living creatures — facts entirely incompatible with prevailing ideas and teachings. But these facts were not only intrinsically veracious but were capable of occular demonstration, beyond all possibility of doubt, and thus, as nothing could be changed or refuted, *science found itself compelled, for once, to honour the truth in its initial stage* — to receive them gracefully unto itself and adopt them in its teachings.

This discovery of the X-rays was followed closely by that of the N-rays, by the two Curies, husband and wife. This further discovery was a still greater surprise to the scientific world than the former one; for by its aid was established nothing less than the inconstancy of matter. Hitherto science, dealing not with knowledge, but with opinions, had held the belief that the atom is the ultimate form of matter and that no chemical or physical force can divide it, a teaching held to be incontrovertible.

First, the discovery of the X-rays had markedly disturbed this belief, and then, on the discovery of the N-rays, it soon became indubitably clear that a constant destruction is taking place within the atom, an uninterrupted throwing off of smaller particles.

But it is not our task to show how one discovery after another was made. We are merely interested in knowing that, because of these discoveries, we find today in the atom — not in the radium atom alone, but in every atom as such — only a union of particles identical with one another, the so-called electrons, being but special forms of electro-magnetic forces.

Professor Gruner writes as follows: "The atom is no longer the accepted, final unit of matter, but has given place to the electron.

The atom is no longer an individual compact particle of matter, but an aggregate of thousands of tiny bodies.

Furthermore, the atom is not indestructible; it can throw off successive electrons or groups of electrons from its numerous contents and so keep up a gradual, but veritable destruction."

Professor Thomson, who won the "Nobel" prize for his work on natural science, makes these distinct assertions:

"(1) The electron is nothing more than a form of electricity.

(2) Each electron weighs 1/770th of a fluid atom. Of an atom, that is, which, hitherto had been regarded as the smallest individual particle.

(3) A fluid atom consists of 770 electrons and is formed of electricity without any other material.

(4) The atoms of other elements, besides radium, are also composed of electrons and of nothing else.

The number of electrons varies in different elements; for instance, an atom of quicksilver is composed of 150,000 electrons.

(5) Electricity is the basis of all being."

Hitherto we have been taught to consider our bodies and their organs from no other standpoint than that of their elements. For if we attribute all the life of the body to the cells, these must consist only of primary matter, like the atoms of which they are formed. But we have now come to know that atoms, and, therefore, our bodies as well, are formed of electrons, or we might say, of crystalized electricity, consequently, we are compelled to recognize in the body a human machine operated entirely under the direction of electrical forces. For electrons cannot lose their electrical character, merely because they are grouped together in atoms and form our bodies.

It is a well known scientific fact that atoms attract and repel each other, just as is the case with electro-magnetic forces.

Our bodies, then, are not only formed of electrons, which unite into atoms, but they are absolutely filled with free electrons; for every atom is surrounded with an envelope of free electrons, or, in other words, is the centre of a molecule of electrons, and carries its envelope of electrons precisely as the earth carries its envelope of air.

Thomson asserts on the basis of his latest observations that:

"Every atom forms a planetary system.

The 150,000 electrons of mercury, for instance, are arranged in four concentric spheres, like a system about the sun."

When we arrive at a complete understanding of these facts and their bearing upon life, we shall be able to control our bodies with perfect success by regulating their electric forces and adjusting their energies.

As yet the main difficulty which obstructs our comprehension comes from the seeming dissimilarity of things within and things without man's "passing strange, complex mortality." This apparent lack of co-ordination presumedly stands in direct contradiction to the similarity of electrons.

But however similar electrons may be, they still have different vibrations, which cause the differences between various objects, — between colors, shapes and sounds, between positive and negative conditions.

It is only by differences of vibration in this world substance, which we may now venture to term electrons, that we are able to perceive a difference in objects around us.

It is a matter of primary interest that the organs of the body should differ in this way; for in them are electrons with their inherent electro-magnetic properties, upon which the whole bodily machinery depends.

Within our bodies positive currents of energy flow from above downward; for manifestly the remainder of the body is governed by the head.

The electrons of the head must consequently be arranged as in a magnet — the positive pole above, the negative below — and they must be always connected with their opposite pole, because the strength and the nature of a magnet depend entirely upon such connection. Thus our heads, under normal conditions, are cool, and our feet warm, so long as positive electro-magnetic force flows from above downward.

In most men of the present day, on the contrary, a condition usually exists the exact opposite of that common to normal healthy individuals.

A sense of well-being prevails in the body only so long as the electrons are in sympathetic contact with their opposite poles, and, because by this means they increase and extend their forces reciprocally, there exists also throughout the entire body a feeling of physical strength.

Life upon the earth is dependent, as we know, upon the power of the sun. Positive electrical forces are displayed in sunlight, and we find that the electrical forces of the soil furnish their complements. Electrical power is manifested by both the earth and the sun—a fact unquestioned by those acquainted with observations made in the field of radio-activity.

As a third factor, absolutely essential, I may mention the ocean, which I regard as the storage battery that distributes the power.

Then mark the natural contrast between these mundane and solar forces—the one of a nature warm and vibrating quickly, the other cold and more slow of vibration.

From this we may infer that we have before us an electrical opposition, a polarity; and assuredly the electrical forces of the earth are those which are negative, since they vibrate more slowly and yield to control, while those of the sun are, on the contrary, positive, since they possess the higher capacity for vibration and dominate the electrical forces of the earth.

We may assert, further, that the forces of the earth are electrical, whilst those of the sun are magnetic. In support of this assertion the proof may be advanced that a magnet can raise a heavier load after lying in the sunlight; for the close affinity, between magnetism and sunlight are, in this way incontestably demonstrated.

The interchange of these principles underlies all mundane activity and existence, and upon its cessation life would wholly disappear from the planet.

The various organs of the body, like everything else, fall under the immediate influence of this interchange of polar forces. The same electric or electro-magnetic opposition exists therein as are elsewhere apparent in nature and, for evidence of the same we have not far to seek.

The phenomena occurring in electrolysis — the science of chemical decomposition by galvanic action — are well known.

When a current of electricity passes through a fluid capable of de-composition the acids gather about the positive pole and the alka-lies about the negative pole. We thus detect the exercise of separate activities on the part of the positive and negative electrical forces, — their polarization, — when we notice that alkalies and acids separate upon the application of electrical forces.

Similar conditions exist in our bodies.

They occur in the mucous and serous membranes; for the serous secretions react acid, the mucous ones, alkaline.

The contrast, in anatomical structure, between the mucous and the serous membranes is due to the fact that they line the various organs, respectively, within and without. It also indicates an opposi-tion in their electro-magnetic forces.

These membranes cover, not only the large organs, but also the small ones, to the smallest muscular fibres.

In this way an electro-magnetic contrast exists in every part of the body, and it is this opposition Of forces which keeps the vital ma-chinery of the body in working order.

Electro-magnetic attraction and resistance are the agencies which control metabolism and the action of the organs, so long as bodily strength and healthy blood are maintained. All internal and external stimuli are nothing more than electro-magnetic processes.

Even our bodily temperature, as we commonly think of it under such conditions, resolves itself into electro-magnetic force or its product.

Electricity, magnetism, light, and heat differ only in respect to vi-bration, and are in the final analysis one and the same.

But since our bodies are not cold like the earth or, like its electric forces, vibrate slowly, but are warm and of quick vibration, we are sufficiently assured that they contain, not only the cold electro-magnetic forces, of slow vibration, but also those that are warm and vibrate rapidly. And thus, when a correct relation exists between positive and negative forces — that is to say, between the forces of electricity and magnetism, then only have we normal temperature, *then alone are we normally healthy.*

When we come to enquire into the sources from which the body obtains these forces, there is little to be said. They are well known, can easily be traced, but to the keenest mind of scholarly research their source of origin is still an unturned page.

Of things in the human economy which count, however, first in importance are food and breath; for in every atom of food we eat and every breath of air we breathe there are electrons which enter the body, there to be seized by the attraction of electro-magnetic action, stored away, and applied in vital processes.

A source of vital energy, commonly known and little recognized, is the free, pure air, or, ether charged with the electrons of space.

Out of space, positive and negative electrons constantly pass into the human body, their effect we feel at once; when, for instance, in a cold room, we commence to feel chilly, or on removal to a warm room, or into the sunlight, a comfortable feeling of warmth pervades the body and restores its normal temperature.

Weather and local conditions have no small influence upon our state of health. In dry and elevated positions or in warm weather the condition of the body is more positive; in damp, low-lying places and in raw weather the electro-magnetic forces have a negative tendency. *This is the explanation of those disturbances of health which occasionally arise and which we sometimes experience in the dire form of epidemics.*

As an illustration, the difference of climatic conditions between the adjoining States of Washington and Oregon are a case in point.

Among other disturbing influences which effect the electro-magnetic forces of the body are *overfeeding* and *underfeeding, too much* and *too little exercise*, particularly too much or too little *stimulation*, or *false stimulation*, or excitement of a physical or mental nature. Any one of these influences may produce disorder in the relations of the electro-magnetic forces of the body. The positive or negative electrons may be abnormally increased or diminished or their location disturbed.

When the body contains too many negative, slowly vibrating forces, or electrons, and its aggregate of electron vibration is consequently diminished, the result follows that the feeling of strength — the vitality, that is, becomes depressed; we feel weak, tired in the limbs; we possess little warmth and easily grow cold; metabolism falls below the normal; the skin becomes pale and so causes the overplus of negative electrons stored in the mucous membrane to set up a morbid action of that structure. Catarrh sets in. In short, negative diseases are the immediate result; such, for example, as nervous debility, anaemia, diabetes, catarrh of the stomach, intestines or air passages, *influenza*, cholera and diphtheria. In these conditions the principles of physiological chemistry laid down by me may well be called into service and improvement effected by a correct adjustment of diet.

When there is an excess of rapidly vibrating, positive electrical forces, or electrons, raising the vitality of the nerves and blood above the normal, the sufferer becomes easily excitable; the body is hot and inclines to inflammatory, feverish or positive diseases, which take the form of inflammation of the lungs, measles, scarlet fever, chicken-pox, typhoid fever, etc.

As I have already remarked, in order to understand a disease and to undertake its cure, it is first of all necessary to form a clear mental picture of its course and origin. With this purpose in view and a medical library at command I have honestly tried to formulate from the initial stages a mental picture of scarlet fever, measles, and kindred ailments; but the entire medical literature did not advance me further than pathological anatomy, which informs us that the original cause of disease is certain changes in the form of the cellular elements of different digestive organs, in the explanation of which the customary technical terms are used, such as atrophy, degeneration and metamorphosis.

By the aid of true physiological chemistry I have been enabled to trace these mysterious incidences in the life current, learning that the cellules — the smallest elements in the human system — require for their composition alternating quantities of different chemical substances.

Which of the chemical elements these are, what mutual relations exist between different organs of the body, and by what means they enter the organism, it has become my intricate and absorbing task to observe.

In this investigation it was gradually made clear to me that every organ and every tissue is dependent upon the introduction of proper nutritive constituents into the blood.

Healthy blood formation is the one great essential requisite to the maintenance of health or the cure of disease. And such blood must be formed from a full supply of the requisite chemical factors, including all of the mineral ingredients.

Dech-Manna Diet.

This is a point commonly overlooked, and my organic nutritive cell-food termed Dech-Manna-Diet is especially designed for the purpose of its enforcement.

In order to obtain a clear understanding of the various forms of disease which attack the human body, it is requisite to know more of the condition we call inflammation. To this end we may consider successively the following facts; namely, that electrons so fill the body as to bring its condition to one equivalent to that of a magnet; that electron lies ranged beside electron; and, that no alteration of location takes place.

Effect of Injury.

But now, suppose some part of the body is subjected to a morbid irritation by some injury. The affected electrons are set into increased vibration and acquire an excess of force above that of the neighbouring electrons. For, the faster a substance vibrates, the more its force increases—a fact with which we are familiar in the action of boiling water and the generation of steam. In proportion as the affected part exceeds the adjoining parts in the vibration of its electrons, it becomes more positive than they and gradually involves these adjoining electrons in the accelerated process of vibration. So, at the seat of injury a centre of positive action is brought into existence which becomes the more intense the longer it continues.

Since the electrons in this locality fall out of their regular positions, in consequence of the general attraction and gravitate toward their appropriate poles, they are found to exercise a reciprocally repellent influence upon each other, by which action the vibration naturally increases still further. This causes pain; for the pronounced opposition of the electrons is attended by a feeling of considerable unpleasantness. The blood, which is an efficient conductor of electro-magnetic force, becomes involved through its ready mobility. The affected part becomes filled with blood. It swells and becomes inflamed;—quickened metabolism and greater warmth are produced by the increase in blood contents and by the more rapid vibrations of the electrons. If the inflammatory process progresses further, the tissues finally disintegrate, partly because of blood stagnation, but chiefly because of the supra-normal vibration of the electrons. Either the tissues are shattered by this motion, or melt in the resultant heat. They undergo purulent disintegration, as we may call it.

Bacteria.

Since the cells created are formed of bacteria, that is to say, of vital germs, as the body tissues are of cells, the destruction of the tissues and cells of necessity sets bacteria free; these therefore are not in reality the cause, but the result of disease.

Febrile, or Positive Diseases.

In pronounced inflammation the disturbance of the electrons, the heat, apart from the functional irregularities which occur in systemic processes, is diffused through the entire body: the sickness becomes fever. The blood is impelled with increased pressure throughout the whole body. If during this process negative electrons hold the preponderance in the body, the fever is of a feeble, adynamic type. But when there are many positive electrons in the body and extensive regions are involved in the disease process, so that pronounced cause exists for increased vibration of electrons, there arise those conditions we designate as scarlet fever, measles, and chicken-pox. For, just as in a steam engine, the increased vibration of the steam exerts a strong pressure upon the piston, so the increased vibration of the electrons in the body finally drives the blood with a similar pressure to the skin, where it produces stasis, or stagnation, sweats and other like disturbances.

Curative Process.

As to curative measures, the course to be followed is clearly self-evident and defined. It could not be other than that of regulating each vibratory body, of soothing the electrons quickened by morbid conditions, and accelerating those which have been depressed.

Law of opposites.

Since treatment can effect this end in no other way than by producing contrary conditions it is evident that a plan of opposition must be followed. And, just as day is the opposite of night, summer of winter, heat of cold, the positive of the negative, so, from the changes effected by this opposition every circumstance and every manifestation takes its rise. This is Natural Law, fixed and immutable throughout nature and for all time. Following this law consistently, our course is clear and simple: in cases of innutrition we seek to increase the nutritive faculty by means of proper food; for the overworked we prescribe rest, for those who need exercise, work; warmth for the cold and cooling for the feverish.

Action of Water.

For cooling we use pure water, the most common and most serviceable of remedies. It cools, soothes and restores equilibrium because its mineral affinities determine its vibratory action as of lower, slower grade, and because one of its constituents is oxygen, the most negative of all elements.

Action of earth or mud.

Even more opposed to inflammation than water, is earth, or mud. Mud produces a more decided cooling effect than water; necessarily so, since its nature is more pronouncedly negative, its vibrations slower. Antiphlogistine, clay acetate, or mud, would be of undoubted service in accordance with the law we have been following; But the same object may be more easily and readily attained by the use of packs.

Vinegar packs.

In employing vinegar in this connection, it should only be used with mud or water. Acids are decidedly negative in their electrical action, and therefore, have a curative effect upon inflammatory diseases. The use of vinegar in connection with clay and water in the treatment of inflammations and fevers is a common, old-time custom; but those who do so, ignorantly perhaps, from force of example or hear-say, unconsciously carry out in so doing one of the plainest scientific laws. Why so? Is it because this liquid kills bacilli or destroys morbid products? No, because it quiets the agitated electrons and equalizes their distribution.

The safest plan is to take two parts water and one part of vinegar. Vinegar prevents coagulation of the blood-cells, and in consequence, stagnation and inflammation are avoided.

Cooling Drinks.

For a similar reason acid drinks, such as lemonade, raspberry vinegar, and diluted raspberry juice, are of the greatest services in inflammations and fevers. They compose the system from within outward. For, as soon as any electrical negative is brought into contact with the system, streams of electricity course through the body and reduce the inflammation. The best lemonade for this purpose is my preparation "Tonogen," because it contains all the necessary acids, besides the necessary constituents for inducing circulation and thereby preventing stagnation It is easily established that patients treated according to my method have become very much stronger and healthier than they were before the beginning of their illness.

Formerly, the proportion of deaths among these who contracted typhoid fever reached twenty and thirty per cent and even higher. These deaths occurred simply because of excessive internal heat. Today, a wide experience shows that hardly any of such cases succumb.

Temperature Reduction.

The application of water in typhoid fever has secured for it a permanent place in the sickroom. Not only have we been enabled by reducing the temperature with water, to attain the very best results in the treatment of typhoid cases, inflammation of the lungs, and all positive heat diseases, but by the same measures, we are now able to forestall its development with increasing certainty.

Brand kept typhoid fever away from his soldiers while it raged around them in the severest form, by the simple specific of a daily bath of an hour's duration in cold water.

It is easy to understand why scarlet fever, measles and chicken-pox—all positive diseases—demand the exclusion of sunlight in their treatment. Experience has shown that the treatment of these diseases makes a more favorable progress when sunlight is excluded.

This fact stands in sharp contrast to all previous observations as to the importance of sunshine in the treatment of disease.

Negative Diseases.

Now let us leave the consideration of the febrile or positive diseases and turn to those of negative character, as well as to disturbances where a reduced vibration of the electrons, a preponderance of cold negative electrical forces, and unhealthy action on the part of the mucous membranes, constitute the condition.

Curative Process.

In this instance, in order to initiate the curative process it is necessary to accelerate the vibration of the electrons in the body — to render the system positive.

The principal remedy is heat, because it engenders a higher rate of vibration of the electrons. For this reason steam baths and other methods of applying heat prove highly remedial in negative diseases of the catarrhal and kindred varieties. They increase the vibration of electrons throughout the body and consequently, stimulate metabolism. The morbid activity of the mucous membranes is reduced and the blood flows actively again toward the surface, so that the internal organs experience immediate relief from abnormal pressure.

Sun baths. Light baths.

Unquestionably in this age, marked as it is by the prevalence of negative ailments, sun baths and electric light baths will celebrate triumph upon triumph over disease, for they reanimate the vibration of the electrons even more than do steam baths, and create a direct supply of rapidly vibrating positive electrons. One can easily be satisfied on this point by observing the result of the simple but conclusive experiment of lying in the sunshine when cold. Baths in electric light and in sunshine strengthen the system of one negatively sick, just as a strong current of inductive electricity gives augmented force to a machine operated by inadequate electric power. The responsive reaction need cause no surprise, for every popular sea-beach shows with what wonderful electrical results a salt water bath is attended when followed by a sun bath in the sand.

.

Exercise.

Equally important in the management of negative diseases is exercise.

Everyone knows that exercise makes us warm, and we know now that warmth comes from a quicker vibration of ether, or rightly speaking, the electrons of ether. So, not only is the circulation of the blood improved and metabolism increased by exercise, above all, the vibration of the electrons is enlivened, thus causing their character to be changed to positivity, and the number of positive electrons in the body to be increased. Consequently, negative diseases, which result from a preponderance of negative electrons in the body, disappear before systematic exercise, as the darkness of night before the rising of the sun.

Massage.

Massage not only removes mechanical disturbances of circulation, but also increases the vibration of electrons in the body. It is, therefore, an invaluable remedy in negative diseases.

In case of chronic depression, we should by no means underestimate the importance of that comfortable feeling induced by the exercise of electronal vibrations, which supervenes upon properly administered massage.

Colored Light Treatment.

A recent method of treatment is that by colored light. Sunshine, prismatically dissected, is known to vibrate at a rate of about four hundred million for red and eight hundred million for blue. The different rays of sunlight therefore must have different effects upon the world of living things, and red light must produce conditions of less violent vibration, blue light of quickened vibration.

In scarlet fever, measles, and chicken-pox, as in all positive febrile diseases, we have seen that there is a morbid increase of vibration in the electrons. Here, therefore, red light is used for curative purposes because it vibrates quietly. In lupus, chronic rheumatism, anemia, and such diseases, a slow vibration of electrons takes place in the body; hence, in such cases, blue light is a medium of cure.

Internal Treatment.

These considerations of the effects of colored light bring us to the treatment of disease by so-called internal means.

Salts.

In a chemical sense the salts of the body are those compounds which consists of two elements, such as water. All salts possess the peculiarity of producing electrical excitation; consequently it is possible for them to generate electricity when coming in contact with carbohydrates. Now the entire structure of the human connective tissue is nothing more or less than a combination of carbohydrates with a salt, that is, with sulphate of lime-ammonia. In this way, natural electrical energy of a positive character exists in the connective tissue which forms the basis of the spleen, the lungs, the stomach, the intestines, the muscles, in fact of the whole body. Therefore, the nervous and arterial systems, together with the heart, are supplied, through the medium of their basis of connective tissues, with electrical energy, by the contact of the electro-negative oxygen which the blood furnishes and the positive sulphate of lime-ammonia in the walls of these organs.

Nourishment.

We now come to a consideration of nourishment. We recognize today the truth of what was asserted years ago by Jezek; namely, that food undergoes a kind of gaseous decomposition in our bodies — one in which the atoms of the elements are resolved into electrons and so become the foundation of new atomic structures. For the separation of atoms into electrons and their entrance into new and different forms — that process which is constantly taking place before our eyes in the external world of Nature — must assuredly be likewise going on in like manner in the human body.

Food.

The world is just awakening and far more inquiry will now be made in the future as to the chemical properties of food, and also as to its necessary quantity and calorific value. It will then be clearly appreciated that vegetable food has a higher value as a producer of energy than animal food, because we find in it in more available form the original elements of force which exists in all matter. For the animal kingdom lives upon the vegetable kingdom and obtains every power it has from vegetable atoms. In the vegetable kingdom the vibration of the electrons is of an electrical character; therefore, vegetable food is of value in the form of electrical force, through its nutritive salts. By maintaining vital processes through its vibrations it renders us another service of a magnetic nature. It is definitely known that quite as much force is derived from vegetable as from animal food, because the former is introduced into the system chiefly in the form of a rapidly vibrating positive magnetic force. Because of its slow vibration vegetable food manifests a lower degree of heat than animal food, and plants possess less warmth than animals.

Diet.

For this reason vegetable diet is distinctly appropriate in febrile diseases. By reason of its more moderate vibration it is also the best diet for nervous people.

Food Standard.

The usefulness of any article of diet depends upon its adaptability for entering into combinations within the system. This, in turn, depends solely upon its higher or lower standing in respect to vibrations. This is the reason why the human organism cannot subsist upon mineral food.

Heat.

We need in our vital economy a definite amount of heat, or positive magnetic force. This is lacking when the system neither produces enough to meet its needs in compensation for expended energy or is not properly supplied with food, fresh air and sunshine.

Discretion.

For this reason it is well to remember that discretion must be used, as any unauthorized, unwise or too rapid change to a strict vegetarian diet may result, in certain cases, in bringing about an underfed condition or in weakening, and even disease, so that the system may be obliged to call in the aid of digestive tonics in order to obtain all the material it needs for the formation of its body-cells.

Enough, however, has been said on the subject I think, to clear the stage, as it were, of the debris of antiquated "orthodox" performances.

We of the independent and rational branch of the science of healing, ignorantly termed "unorthodox," have devised a means of preventing disease and curing it, when encountered, in a natural way, with materials that regenerate and invigorate the blood, and this method is slowly but surely fighting its way into general recognition. In time we may hope to be able to make the so-called "inevitable" children's complaints a matter of the past, and to raise a generation in which the sins of the forefathers shall be extinct, so that sane and healthy offspring will be the result. But pending such time — until the final victory of the biological-hygienic system for the prevention of disease — we are now prepared and able to cope with the still existing conditions, and to heal, if proper attention is paid to our teachings.

Diet for Children in General.

For the infant child as well as for its mother, it is naturally best that it should be nursed by the mother. The infant should receive the breast every three hours approximately, and no food should be given it during the night, in order to make the feeding regular and avoid intestinal catarrh through overfeeding.

A regular diet is necessary for a nursing mother. Hot spices and foods producing gas, must be avoided. Tight clothes that cause degeneration of the mammary glands, are prohibited.

If the mother is unable to nurse the child, and a wet-nurse cannot be afforded, the child must be fed artificially, and this requires painstaking care and attention.

The main factor is to secure good cow's milk, which is most like human milk. Milk from cows that are kept in barns, should not be used, for these animals constantly live in stables that lack fresh air, and under conditions very detrimental to the milk.

The milk should be warmed carefully, thereby approximating the temperature of the mother's milk (86° to 98.6°) before it is given to the infant. The nursing bottle and the rubber caps must be kept scrupulously clean. The milk should be shaken thoroughly before being used, in order to make a perfect intermixture of milk and cream.

The newly born infant is not able to digest undiluted milk, and therefore must receive:

1st to 5th day: 1 part milk to three parts water.

5th to 30th day: 1 part milk to two parts water.

30th to 60th day: Half milk, half water.

3rd to 8th month: I part milk, one-half part water.

Or:

1st to 3rd month, every 2 hours; 1 part milk, two parts water, with the addition of 2 table-spoonsful milk sugar to I or 1½ quarts milk.

4th to 5th month, every 3 hours: 1 part milk, 1 part water.

6th to 9th month: 2 parts milk, 1 part water.

Thereafter pure milk, with the addition of very little sugar, or gruel made of oatmeal or something similar. Among the preparations that are best known are Knorr's and Nestle's.

Not until the first teeth have made their appearance, should the child begin to have thin groat soup, a few soft boiled eggs, and a little more solid food.

Infants fed artificially must receive food frequently.

Later on, still maintaining the milk diet, light milk and flour food, vegetables and meat gravy may be given. Infants and even older children should, under no circumstances, receive miscellaneous delicacies, or highly seasoned and greasy dishes. Strong tea and coffee are poison to the nervous system of children.

In case of intestinal diseases milk must be substituted for other diet, with decoctions of cereal flour. Furthermore, Dech-Manna chocolate and malt-chocolate, boiled in milk, are recommended.

Diet for School Children.

The appetite of children increases with their growth and years, and is always a sign of good health. Much exercise in the open air is of the greatest benefit to children. It is not, however, immaterial how children are fed. The theory that children should receive whatever is served on the family table, may be correct from the standpoint of discipline, but it may bring about trouble if the food that is offered does not agree with the stomach of the child. Food for children should be light and display variety. It is not correct to believe that what is eaten with aversion, has a healthy effect, and by forcing children to eat food against which their natural instinct rebels, parents have often seriously injured their children.

In a general way, soup, vegetables, farinaceous food or a little meat and fruit is sufficient for the principal meal.

In the morning a cup of milk, cocoa or weak coffee (fruit or malt), with a piece of bread; for anaemic children, butter and bread and honey. Prepared in various forms, plenty of milk and farinaceous food, rice, groat, oats, barley, cornmeal, fruit and cooked fruit should be eaten, which all children like and which are superior in effect, since they are so easily digested. Pure water with a little fruit-juice added occasionally; in the afternoon weak tea with milk, fruit coffee, cocoa, malt chocolate; in the summer time, cold sweet or sour milk; these should be the drinks for growing children. Bread and butter with a little marmalade is always welcome. When fruit is in season, some fresh fruit and dry bread is sufficient in the afternoon; the supper should be simple, warm or cold, but without high seasoning; potatoes with butter, soft boiled eggs, bread and ham, cold roast meat, soup or some well prepared farinaceous food one hour before bedtime. Food should not be served very hot, should be well masticated and eaten with little to drink during the meal. It is better to take a glass of water before the meal.

Alcoholic drinks are strictly prohibited, since they produce nervous irritation and make study much harder.

Game, when not too high and without spice is good for growing children. Dishes prepared from internal organs, such as liver, kidneys and brains, are usually repugnant to children, and should be avoided. Steamed vegetables are preferable to those cooked with sauce. Salads for children should not be highly seasoned, but should be prepared with butter, cream and lemon juice, in which form they are of great nutritive value. Avoid delicacies and mayonnaise dressing. Ice cream is the delight of most children. Permit small quantities, but eaten with crisp biscuit only, so as to avoid catarrh of the stomach.

Children should have one or two meals between the regular meals. Greatest variety should prevail at dinner and supper, and the favorite dishes of the various children should be served from time to time.

Taste and appetite are the means by which the intestinal organs express what they consider most suitable for the system. That which tastes good not only influences the health of the body, but also the mental condition of the child. Proper food, ample time for play and much fresh air will make the physician's visit a rare necessity. However, if a child becomes ill, medical advice should be obtained immediately and followed strictly, thus avoiding many sad experiences.

Nearly all forms of children's disease are combined with fever, and even without any of the characteristic symptoms of the various forms of disease, children are often subject to more or less intense attacks of fever. Therefore, in the following pages I am giving an extensive description of fever from a biological standpoint, together with its dietetic treatment—not *cure* for, as will be seen, *fever in itself is not a disease, but the attempt of nature to get rid of a disease.*

This elaborate description of fever in all its phases will also serve as a valuable illustration of the manner in which all subjects dealt with are treated in my greater work: "Regeneration, or Dare to be Healthy."

FEVER AND ITS TREATMENT, BASED ON BIOLOGY
(A) GENERAL DESCRIPTION.

Fever is one of the protective institutions of the body, which very often acts most advantageously in the interests of the preservation of the organism. It is a symptom, or rather a group of symptoms, consisting of an increase of temperature, acceleration of metabolism, excitement of the nerves, numbness and frequently delirium.

Undoubtedly a fever of long duration and high temperature may injure the organism to the extent that death ensues.

There have been, nevertheless, at all times, those who hold the opinion that fever, as such, does not under any circumstances, injure the organism of itself alone.

Fever has at all times been regarded, and to a much higher degree today than formerly, as a healthy reaction against diseased matter, and indeed, as an expression of the healing tendency of nature, Hippocrates considered it an excellent remedy. Thomas Campanello recognized its qualities of removing diseased matter.

This doctrine is corroborated by the findings in regard to infections.

Through fever the organism is freed from micro-organisms which may have forced their way in. Fever operates like fire, destroying the contagious matter. After this is done the remnants are excreted through intense and extremely offensive perspiration.

Experiments have taught us that the growth and the resisting power of many microbes decrease if the temperature of the body rises, but 1.8 to 3.6 degrees above normal. It is also a remarkable fact that in every disease where bacteria are found, there is a special type of fever, which takes its course in such strict accordance with its law, that the physician is thereby able to determine the nature of the disease.

While the degree of temperature is decisive in regard to the life of micro-organisms, the height of the temperature does not, in itself, constitute a criterion of the gravity of danger. It is the duty of the physician to fight the fever, since the patient may succumb to a high temperature, as to a low one.

In order to gauge the situation accurately it is necessary to regard fever, not as a disease, but as what it really is in essence: a symptom which accompanies the greatest variety of the processes of disease, — symptom of the most variable significance in various cases. It must be fought like other symptoms, such as vomiting, coughing, pains and diarrhoea; namely, in a general way — provided only that it is not a manifestation of the healing tendency of the organism.

In decreasing the fever, we moderate the excitement of the nerves, remove the numbness, secure calmness, refreshment and sleep, and defend the patient against threatening manifestations of disease.

Very often it is not a case of treating the fever, but of dealing with the disease which causes the fever. We must consequently not be guided by the thermometer but by the condition of the nervous system.

Two conditions must be observed in treating fever according to the rules of biology.

In the first place, the treatment of febrile disease must not be carried on in accordance with general principles, but individually, according to the nature of the disease in each particular case.

In the second place, it is necessary that the antipyretic treatment, to reduce the fever, should not be foreign to the organism and should not be such as is not measurable in degrees as to its effects, or has any unpleasant accompanying effects or after-effects.

Only the biological system of healing responds to these demands. Only cognate physical forces, in affinity with the human organism according to biological laws, can influence vital occurrences with the hope of success and without the danger of unfavorable accompanying effects and consequences.

Only physical remedies and treatments permit of adequate gradations such as will appeal to the power of reaction of the organism.

In the appropriate application of certain, influences of nature, especially in the diversified applications of water, we possess a mode of procedure which, assisted by an appropriate dietetic regime adapted to the principles of biological healing and to the conditions of life in health and disease, offers advantages which no other treatment affords and benefits the patient to an extent which cannot be too highly estimated.

In the treatment of fever we must, in the first place, follow the impulses of instinct—harmonized, however, with the fundamental laws and methods of biological treatment—if success is to be obtained. Instinctively, in the case of a hot forehead, we turn to the application of cold compresses; for cold feet, the use of such appliances as will bring about heat. Tormenting thirst is assuaged by a mouthful of cooling water. But the instinct of impulse alone might also lead one burning with high fever to seek relief by immersion in cooling water; thus, in order to discover the rational course we must be guided by the fundamental laws of the biological system of healing.

(B) TREATMENT.

To these biological explanations of what fever is, it will be interesting to add some general description and explanation of its treatment, such as may serve in an emergency as an indication of the proper course to be pursued and by the most simple means, pending the attendance of an hygienic physician.

I must again call special attention to the importance of not clinging too literally to the letter of the law,—of every rule laid down,—but rather to study by the light of such laws and with alert intelligence the special features of the case at issue.

Of all hygienic treatments of fever, which have come under my notice in the course of many years, there is none more clearly, simply and intelligibly described than that which Dr. C. Sturm, has published in his book, "Die natur liche Heilmethode" (The Natural Method of Healing). I will, therefore, employ it in my explanations, (as translated from the German) adding to it my advanced methods, especially the hydropathic and dietetic treatments which are more in accordance with the demands of modern biological therapy.

In the first place, as we know, fever is indicated by an abnormally hot skin. This heat is noticeable even by touching the patient with the palm of the hand.

A precise measurement of this heat, of course, requires a thermometer. The best kind is a so-called maximum thermometer.

The temperature is taken by putting the lower end of the glass into the axilla, or arm-pit, of the arm, or in the mouth or the rectum of the patient, and leaving it there for from 8 to 10 minutes. When withdrawn, the temperature of the patient can be read at a glance.

The temperature of the skin, however, is not the only indication of fever. It is accompanied simultaneously by accelerated action of the pulse, up to 120 beats per minute, and even more; also by increased thirst and, as an indication of very intense affection, extreme exhaustion and lassitude. The increased excretion becomes manifest through dark and strong-smelling urine and, especially at the time when the fever begins to abate, through intense perspiration.

In the beginning of fever the change alternating between chills and abnormal heat is very characteristic; frequently, and especially in severe attacks, it begins with shivers. The patient suddenly feels an intense chill, so that he commences to shake all over, his teeth chatter and he grasps whatever covering he can for warmth. Suddenly, following this, a rapid increase of temperature occurs, and the patient begins to complain of intense heat. In other cases patients complain of feeling very cold, while their skin indicates a marked degree of warmth.

With higher degrees of temperature, the fever may induce a loss of consciousness. The patient becomes delirious, loses urinary and fecal control and displays the signs of total collapse.

Fever, as I have already indicated, is a kind of physical revolution, a state of excitation which, differing so widely as to cause, character and degree, cannot be judged according to any fixed rule. The temperature of a patient we may read from the thermometer; but the real nature of the fever we do not learn until we consider his constitution, his innate faculties and the strength to which his various organs have attained. For this purpose we must take into consideration not only the physical attributes, but also the quality of the senses and of the mind, since these items are of the utmost importance in determining the tenacity, i.e., the power of resistance of the patient.

From this point of view it will be understood that people possessing a calm and phlegmatic temperament, will not attain to high degrees of fever, except in cases of very serious complications, while nervous people may quickly reach very considerable degrees of temperature. Children and younger people are more inclined to high fever, since their organs are still immature. This explains why simple inflammations, which are not general throughout the body, or frequent indigestion, which in itself does not figure as a dangerous illness, will in the case of children appear under the gravest symptoms. It follows, therefore, how necessary it is to discriminate closely and decide accordingly between severe symptoms of fever as manifested by people of calm temperament, and similar cases when manifested by people of nervous temperament.

Unfortunately fever has been treated in the past according to set and rigid rules. As soon as the temperature of a patient rose from 98.6° and 99.6° to 100.4°, it was pronounced to be fever, and preparations were made to treat it accordingly. The treatment became more energetic the higher the fever rose to 105.8° and 107.6°.

It was said that under all circumstances the temperature must be lowered to normal.

This idea is decidedly wrong and most dangerous for the patient. For, while a calm and phlegmatic patient may withstand this strong reduction of excitement in his internal organs, which in fact require it, the procedure necessary to bring it about, as a rule exceeds what the nervous patient can endure.

The fever should only be reduced in accordance with the strength of the patient, otherwise extreme irritation must ensue, such as has caused the death of hundreds of thousands in the past. It is better, therefore, to leave a nervous patient in his fever and strengthen him by various devices, so that he may overcome it. Later he may require and, consequently, be able to withstand stronger measures. For this purpose I recommend simple ablutions, in some cases the application of abdominal packs for half an hour *using two-thirds water and one-third vinegar*, as previously prescribed. In addition, the natural vigor of the patient is to be strengthened by administering to him, at intervals of from half an hour to two hours, Dechmann's Tonogen and Dechmann's Plasmogen alternately.

The treatment must be in proportion to the strength of the patient. Thus the quiet, energetic temperament can endure more extensive packs; his nature in fact requires them. His body may be completely packed or at least three-quarters, by placing the moist sheet around his entire body except the arms, while the woolen blanket is either wrapped around the whole body, including the arms, or, as before, leaves the patient free to move his arms, which are then only covered by the bed-clothes. A patient of this kind may also be treated with ablutions or put into a half bath at 75.2°, while cooler water is poured over him. Young and strong patients have endured even cooler baths as powerful stimulants.

The nearer a patient approaches to a nervous, weak condition, the more caution is required to allow him hike warm baths only, or, still better, ablutions at 77°, which may be made severer by not drying the patient.

It is very beneficial to weak patients to frequently wash their hands, face and neck, without drying them.

A very careful treatment of the hair is also a great necessity, especially for women. Clean and well combed hair is very beneficial to a patient. Slight ablutions of the head and combing the hair while wet, are very cooling and refreshing.

The stronger the nature of a patient, the safer it becomes to rely upon a single mode of procedure. Thus, cold packs may be sufficient in case of high fever if applied about every half hour or hour; or, if the temperature is not quite so high, at intervals, from one hour and a half to two hours With weaker persons more variety of procedure is imperative, but none of them must be too stringently applied. In these cases mild ablutions should be used several times during the day, and they may be alternated with packs of the whole lower part of the body or packs on the calves of the legs.

Cool or cold enemas are rapidly absorbed and thus have a quieting influence on the large blood reservoir in the abdomen. Little mouthfuls of water are also taken from time to time, but too much water always weakens the patient.

(C) DIET IN CASES OF FEVER.

As diet in cases of fever I recommend the prescriptions of Professor Moritz, which coincide with my own experiences, so far as a fever diet is concerned; and in addition the physiologico-chemical cell-food which I have used for many years with the greatest success (Dech-Manna Diet). The importance of the latter is due to the fact that it not only *prevents* the destruction of the cells, but has a general strengthening effect upon the system.

Whatever the differences in manifestation the febrile diseases may show, the *febrile reduction of the digestive capacity of the stomach and the bowels is so characteristic*, that it should be specially noted in this connection.

True, fever shows considerable *disturbance of metabolism*, since the *decomposition of the albumen is increased in an abnormal way*. This fact, however, does not demand any particular attention, in regard to diet. As far as possible during fever it is well to exercise an economizing influence on the decomposition of the albumen of the body through the introduction of *all kinds of food* that produce energy, so that it is not necessary to *give preference to any one particular kind of food*.

The injury to digestion during fever comprises not only the peptic functions, which manifest themselves clearly in a reduction of the excretion of hydrochloric acid, but all functions pertaining thereto, the motory as well as the resorptive.

The danger that the patient will receive too much solid food, hard to digest, is generally speaking not very great since, during acute fever, patients as a rule show a decided lack of appetite. The other extreme is the more likely to occur; that the amount of nutrition given may be less than what is requisite and helpful; too much deference being paid to the inclinations of the patient. Formerly the general belief obtained that fever would be increased, in a degree detrimental to the patient, by allowing the consumption of any considerable amount of food, and following this doctrine, the patient was permitted to go hungry. This, however, is absolutely erroneous. *No one would feed a feverish person in a forcible manner, but it is absolutely imperative to take care that he receives food productive of energy in reasonable quantities.*

As a rule hardly one-half, or at the most two-thirds of the normal quantity of nourishment necessary for the preservation of life, may be introduced into the organism in case of acute febrile disease. I have already indicated that there is no particular danger in such partial "inanition" (starvation) for a short period, but that, accordingly, the qualitative side of the nourishment becomes more important the longer the fever lasts. It has also been mentioned that the organism reduces its work of decomposition, gradually adapting itself to the unfavorable conditions of sustenance, and thus meets our efforts to maintain its material equilibrium.

It is important always to make use of any periods of remission and intermission, during which the patient has a better appetite and can digest more easily, to give him a good supply of food. It is also well to administer *as much nourishing food as possible* in the beginning of an illness, which is likely to be lengthy, provided the patient is not yet wholly under the effects of the febrile disease. The food must then be gradually reduced in the course of the illness.

As to quality, the diet must be selected from forms II and III (as below), and will consequently consist of glutinous soups, in some cases with the addition of a nutritive preparation of egg, meat jelly, milk and possibly thin gruel and milk.

The quantity of food which the patient may receive can only be given approximately, as follows:

For adults — (to constitute a sustaining diet). Soup ½ pint, milk and milk gruel ⅓ pint, meat 3 oz., farinaceous food the same, 2 eggs, potatoes, vegetables, fruit sauces 2 to 2½., pastry and bread 2 oz.

These quantities must be considered as the maximum for each portion. The quantity of beverage at each meal must also be very limited, not exceeding 3 to 6 oz., so that the stomach is not overburdened unnecessarily nor its contents too much diluted.

The reduced meals are harmonized with the object of sufficient general nourishment by eating more frequently, about five to six times a day. Patients with fever should have some food in small quantity every 2 to 3 hours. It is important that *the patient be fed regularly at fixed times.* This will be found advantageous both for the patient and for nursing.

Form II comprises *purely liquid nourishment, "soup diet."* Consommé of pigeon, chicken, veal, mutton, beef, beef-tea, meat jelly, which becomes liquid under the influence of bodily heat, strained soups or such as are prepared of the finest flour with water or bouillon, of barley, oats, rice (glutinous soup), green corn, rye flour, malted milk. All of these soups, with or without any additions such as raw eggs, either whole or the yolk only, if well mixed and not coagulated are easily digested. (Besides albumen preparations, Dech-Manna powders, dry extract of malt, etc., may be added).

Form III comprises *nourishment which is not purely liquid.* Milk and milk preparations (belonging to this group on account of their coagulation in the stomach):

(a) — Cow's milk, diluted and without cream, dilution with ½ to ⅔ barley water, rice water, lime water, vichy water, pure water, light tea.

(b) — Milk without cream, not diluted.

(c) — Full milk, either diluted or undiluted.

(d) — Cream, either diluted or undiluted.

(e) — All of these milk combinations with an addition of yolk of egg, well mixed, whole egg, cacao, also a combination of egg and cacao.

Milk porridge made of flour for children, arrowroot, cereal flour of every kind, especially oats, groat soups with tapioca, or sago, and potato soup.

Egg, raw, stirred, or sucked from the shell, or slightly warmed and poured into a cup; all either with or without a little sugar or salt.

Biscuit and crackers, well masticated to be taken with milk, porridge, etc.

As a rule fever is accompanied by an increased thirst, which may be satisfied without hesitation. It is unnecessary, and detrimental, for patients suffering from an increased excretion of water through the fever heat, to be subjected to thirst. Since the mucous membrane of the digestive channel is usually not very sensitive to weak chemical food irritations, the cooling drinks, which contain fruit acids, such as fruit juices and lemonades, are as a rule permissible. Fruit soups may also be given.

It is different, of course, if an acute catarrh of the stomach or of the bowels is combined with the fever. In such cases fruit acids must be avoided. Still it is not necessary to resist the desire of the patient to take whatever may be given him, at a low temperature. Even ice cream, vanilla or fruit water ice, may be used in moderate quantity.

Warning against cold drinks is necessary only in case of disease of the respiratory organs when the cold liquids would cause coughing.

The use of dietetic stimulants such as Dechmann's Tonogen, Eubiogen and Plasmogen, is the same in these cases as has been mentioned in several places previously.

As soon as the patient has made sufficient progress, he may receive more solid food.

The salivary digestion being improved, he may now be allowed several more substantial dishes of rice and groat, cooked partly in milk, partly in water and eaten with fruit juice. He may also have several kinds of green vegetables, like spinach, cauliflower, asparagus, comfrey, etc.

With additional increase in his strength, fresh fish, well prepared, is especially refreshing to a patient with light fever.

As to mental pabulum, in case of severe fever, I recommend for the patient absolute mental and physical rest; little talking, no noise, no visits, no disturbance of any kind. Within his system nature has to accomplish an enormous task to facilitate which complete quiet is essential. Just as he who has serious preoccupations needs quiet environment, so that his attention may be devoted to his thoughts, so also a patient in the throes of fever must relax all external considerations in deference to the struggle of the vital forces within. Whatever disturbance of mentality occurs has always prejudicial effects, such indeed as may in some cases cost the life all are seeking to save.

SCARLET FEVER.

Scarlet fever is an exanthematous form of disease distinguished by a scarlet eruption of the skin. It produces marked symptoms in three localities, the skin the throat and the kidneys.

It is doubtful whether it can be conveyed from one person to another; at least nothing is known concerning the "contagium," or germ of conveyance of infection,—according to the differential diagnosis of Dr. G. Kuhnemann, whose work on the subject is held to be authoritative. It is not to be denied that the disease may be carried by articles of clothing and by intermediary persons, who themselves are not suffering from it.

The incubation period—the time intervening between infection and eruption—during which the infected person is "sickening for" disease, varies from two to as much as eight days.

Chills, feverishness, headache, nausea and actual vomiting are the initial symptoms, and sore throat with difficulty in swallowing soon follow.

Inspection reveals the appearance of an acute throat inflammation, and the tip and sides of the tongue are red as a raspberry. A few hours later—or at most a day or two—the eruption appears; first in the throat, then on the face and chest. It begins with minute, bright red, scattered spots, steadily growing larger until they run together so that the entire skin becomes scarlet, being completely covered with them. Frequently the temperature in the evening ranges as high as from 103° to 105° Fahrenheit. Albumen is always found in the urine.

After two or more days the fever mounts gradually, the throat symptoms increase, the eruption fades away, and from four to eight days later the patient's condition returns to normal.

At the beginning of the second week desquamation, or scaling, begins, the skin peeling off in minute flakes. At this stage heavy sweats set in and the excretion of urine is increased.

In epidemic form the type is sometimes much more malignant, even to the degree that death occurs on the first day with typhoid and inflammatory brain symptoms, unconsciousness, convulsions, delirium, excessive temperature, and rapid pulse. This may happen even without the eruption becoming fairly recognizable. In such severe epidemics the throat symptoms are apt to take on the aspect of diphtheria. The renal discharge exhibits the conditions of a catarrh of the urinary canals originating from causes we do not understand.

Among the after effects of scarlet fever are inflammation of the ear with all its consequences, and inflammatory affections of the lungs, air passages, diaphragm and heart membrane.

The cause, I repeat again, is *dysaemia*—impure blood.

If the patient is predisposed to this form of disease and moreover, a weakling, the case is a dangerous one.

Every good mother should see to it that there is healthy blood in her offspring. The task is comparatively an easy one, the method, is simple and ignorance ceases to be an excuse, for my object is to place the necessary knowledge within the reach of all.

The treatment of scarlet fever varies according to which symptoms are most severe.

In the first place prophylactic efforts must be constantly employed to prevent *possible* contagion. Healthy children must be strictly seperated from the sick till the end of desquamation or scaling—a period of four to six weeks.

If the course of the attack is normal, the patient should be kept in bed under a light cover with a room temperature of 60° to 65°. The sick room must be well ventilated and aired daily.

The windows should be hung with transparent *red* curtains.

The diet may consist of milk, curds, barley soup, oatmeal gruel, flour gruel, with some cooked fruit and, of drinks, lemonade, soda water, and raspberry juice; but the most important drink from a scientific point is Dechmann's "Tonogen," as previously described.

The linen should be changed often

Sponge baths with chilled vinegar-water (1 part cider vinegar diluted with 2 parts water) are helpful when the temperature rises to

102°. If the temperature reaches 105° or over, baths must be promptly administered. The patient may be placed in a bath of 85° or 90°, and the water allowed to cool gradually down to 70° or 65°.

A sick child may stay in such a bath ten or twenty minutes, while the time in a bath practically should not be more than three or five minutes. The bath must be repeated as soon as the fever again reaches 105°.

When the first symptoms of measles, scarlet fever or chicken-pox are noticed, give the child a three-quarter pack. (See directions under "packs"). After each pack sponge the patient with cool vinegar-water.

If the fever is high during the night, apply a sponge bath every half hour or hour.

During the day give the patient ¼ teaspoonful of Dechmann's Plasmogen, dissolved in ½ pint water, a little every hour.

In the evening and during the night alternate this blood-salt solution with Tonogen.

Blood plasm contains eight different salts in different composition, and only when the actual physiological composition is employed can there be any guarantee against the decomposition of the blood-cells. Plasmogen is such a composition.

When diphtheria and Bright's disease complicate the case, they must be dealt with as under ordinary conditions and treated by a competent, Hygienic dietetic physician.

If recovery is prompt and desquamation (scaling) is in progress, warm baths may be applied for a few days.

When the temperature and urine continue normal for a few weeks, the child may be regarded as restored to health.

MEASLES.

Measles or Rubeola is an exanthematous or eruptive contagious form of children's disease.

In Measles the medium of contagion is the excretion from the air passages, mucus coughed up and air exhaled; also the saliva, tears, blood and perspiration of the patient.

In Measles also, as is the case with regard to scarlet fever, the "contagium," or germ of contagion, is unknown.

The general susceptibility to measles is extraordinarily great the poison being of a virulent nature.

If the disease attacks one of feeble constitution whose environment is unfavorable and insanitary,—dwelling in badly ventilated rooms, for instance, with little attention paid to personal cleanliness, the attack is likely to assume a malignant form.

A period of from ten to fourteen days may elapse between infection and the development of the symptoms.

During this period the patient may infect others.

This explains how easily a whole school may become infected.

During the preliminary period children feel tired, relaxed, suffer pain in the joints and headache; they have chills and are feverish at evening. Among the symptoms enumerated are catarrhal affections of the air passages, the larynx, the nose and eyes. Constant sneezing, nosebleeding, cough, watering eyes, ultra sensitiveness to strong light, are concurrent conditions. At the same time the fever becomes pronounced.

These symptoms continue for four or five days and then rapidly abate and the eruption appears. First a red rash is seen, which spreads over the surface of the face. Inside the mouth and throat a similar mottled redness is seen. In the course of a day the eruption spreads over the whole body. After continuing at their height for a day or two the symptoms gradually decline, and in a little over a week the child may be pronounced well. The skin then sheds all the superfluous cuticle left by the eruption, and in three or four weeks after inception the normal condition is again reached.

In the malignant form all the symptoms are of a severe type. Occasionally catarrhal affections of the air passages, croup or pulmonary inflammation supervene, and the patient succumbs.

Other concurrent forms of disease are whooping cough, diphtheria, pulmonary consumption, inflammation of the eyes, ear disease, and swelling of the glands.

Measles demand no distinctive treatment. The room must be well ventilated, with a temperature of about 60°, and light must be almost totally excluded. At night no lamp should be allowed.

Treatment and diet should be the same as in scarlet fever.

GERMAN MEASLES.

German Measles (Rubella or Roetheln), is an eruptive form of children's disease, much more harmless than the disturbances previously depicted. It is one which occurs in epidemics, but to which children individually are largely susceptible; the actual contagium thereof, however, is likewise unknown to science.

Eight days generally intervene between the time of infection and the breaking out of the rash.

During this period no acute symptom is noticeable. In the majority of cases the fever that precedes the eruption is not high; headache, cold and sorethroat accompany the appearances of the rash, which in this case breaks out at once, and not after several days, as in the case of actual measles. The spots are about the size of lentils, and are quite deep red, appearing first upon the face.

After the rash has been out for one or two days, it gradually becomes paler, the fever goes down, and recovery progresses rapidly, usually without any after effects.

It is not necessary for the patient to remain in bed longer than three or four days; nevertheless, the treatment should be just the same as prescribed in the case of the real measles, so as not to leave any weakness or subsequent complication.

There are many other forms of disease, besides these, which are likewise accompanied by fever and a rash, which also appear in epidemics and are evidently due to a great variety of causes. As they, however, invariably run the natural course, I shall not dwell upon them here.

CHICKEN-POX.

Chicken-pox, or Varicella, of which the contagium also remains a mystery, is another infectious eruptive form of disease, peculiar to children. It begins with the appearance of a number of little pigmented elevations on the skin which develop into vesicles and pustules. After a certain period they become encrusted with scabs, which dry up and fall off. When the pustules are deep-seated, small scars remain There is no fever, and the illness is over in about fourteen days. The contagion passes through personal contact, or through clothing and bed linen.

If symptoms are severe enough to require it, treatment should follow the directions for scarlet fever.

SMALL-POX.

As a matter of fact Chicken-pox is of congeneric origin with small-pox, with which, in a very much milder degree, it has various features in common. But small-pox itself is engendered of foul and insanitary conditions of life, impure blood and bad and insufficient nourishment and these, together with its risk under unscientific conditions and in times past of facial disfigurement, have made its name more repugnant to the layman than perhaps any other form of disease. All that need be said about it here, however, is that it is largely a terror of the past and that the sure preventative against it always, and the one reliable anti-toxin against contagion, under all circumstances, is good healthy blood and hygienic-dietetic living.

Those readers who may desire a minute description of this form of disease will find the same in chapt: XII of my greater work "Re-generation."

TYPHOID FEVER OR TYPHUS ABDOMINALIS.

(A) General Description.

This description of fever is usually termed typhus or nerve fever. It characterizes all forms of typhoid disease of which the following features constitute the prominent symptoms.

To a peculiar degree, chiefly young and strong individuals of from 15 to 30 years of age are attacked by this disease, while those in early youth and of more advanced years are much less subject to the same.

It is a complaint very dangerous to those who eat and drink to excess and without discretion. Strong excitement of the mind, such as a shock or great anguish, will undoubtedly favor the appearance of typhus. The seasons too have considerable influence upon it, most cases occurring during the Autumn months—from August to November.

It has been previously indicated to what extent the study of the hygienic conditions of life will assist in the discovery of the real causes of so-called contagious disease. One instance may show the enormous influence of dietetic movements on the outbreak of great epidemics.

It is reported in the "Journal of the Sanitary Institute," London, that the English Seaside Resort Brighton, in the period from July, 1893, to August, 1896, 238 cases of abdominal typhus were observed,—about equally divided for the different years. In 56 cases the typhus was caused by the eating of oysters (36 cases) or clams (20 cases). There was evidence that the water from which these oysters and clams were taken was badly polluted by the excrement of several thousand people, brought through sewers to the place were the shell-fish had been gathered. It was very characteristic in a number of cases that only one of a number of persons, who were otherwise living under equal conditions, fell ill with typhus, a short while after having eaten some of the shell-fish. No other points essential to the spreading of this contagious disease could be discovered. Brighton is healthily situated and built; hygienic conditions in general are favourable; much attention is paid particularly to keeping the soil clean, removing all faeces and providing good drinking water. Contamination through milk in all of the 56 cases, according to most careful investigations, was out of the question. They occurred in entirely different streets in various precincts of the town; 45 of the patients lived on 43 different streets. Besides the people attacked by typhus, many other persons fell ill from lighter disease of the intestines, after having eaten of these crustaceous bivalves, the symptoms being diarrhoea and pains in the stomach. Measures were taken to remove the noxious causes as soon as the source of infection was discovered.

The same conditions were some time ago noticed in Berlin. Out of 14 people invited to a dinner, nine fell ill — 5 of them very serious-ly — under symptoms of typhus, after having eaten oysters from Heligoland. Part of the personnel of the kitchen and some of the servants were taken ill with the same critical symptoms.

B. Essentials.

Abdominal typhus is a general illness of the whole body, and consequently all organs of the body are more or less altered in a morbid way while the disease lasts. The main change occurs in the lymphatic glands of the intestines and in the spleen.

The following are its anatomical symptoms: With the beginning of the disease the lymphatic glands of the mucous membrane of the intestines begin to swell; they are constantly growing during the course of the disease and attain the size of a pea; extended over the level of the mucous membrane they feel firm, hard and tough. In favourable cases the swelling may go down at this stage, but gener-ally the formation of matter begins through the dying of the cells, caused by insufficient nourishment. This is gradually thrown off, and a loss of substance remains — the typhoid ulcer. This varies in size and in depth. Light bleeding in no great quantity ensues. If the ulcer has gone very deep, the intestines may be perforated and then the faeces and part of the food enter the abdominal cavity. The re-sult is purulent and ichorous peritonitis. As a rule, however, the ulcers are purified and heal by cicatrization. Usually the spleen is enormously enlarged (through a rapid increase in the number of its cells). The swelling of the spleen can easily be detected by external touch.

(C) Symptoms and Course.

During what is termed the earlier stage, which as a rule last about two weeks and precedes the breaking out of the disease proper, the patient still feels comparatively well, or only begins to complain of headache, tired feeling, prostration in all the limbs, dizziness, lack of appetite. It is thus absolutely impossible to fix a definite date for its development. In most cases the patient complains of a chill, followed by feverishness, — symptoms which confine him to bed, — although no actual shivering takes place. It is expedient, although quite arbitrary and subject to many modifications, to divide the course of the illness into three periods: —

(1) The stage of development.

(2) The climax.

(3) The stage of healing.

During the stage of development, which usually lasts about a week, the symptoms of the disease rapidly increase. The patient gets extremely weak and faint, has severe headaches and absolutely no appetite. In consequence of the high fever, he complains of thirst; the skin is dry, the lips chapped, the tongue coated; the pulse is rapid and full; the bowels are constipated, but the abdomen is practically not inflated nor sensitive to pressure. In most cases the spleen is evidently enlarged.

Before the end of the first week the climax is reached. This in the lighter cases lasts for the second week, or in more severe cases, even until the third. The fever is constantly high, even 104° and over. The body is generally benumbed, the patient becomes delirious at night or lies absolutely indifferent to all surroundings. The abdomen is now inflated, the buttocks show small, light red spots, — the so-called "roseola," — which are characteristic of abdominal typhus. Furthermore, in most cases, bronchial catarrh of a more or less severe nature appears. Instead of obstruction of the bowels there is diarrhoea — about two to six light yellow thin stools, occur within 24 hours. During this second stage the complications appear.

At the end of the second or the third week respectively, the fever slackens; in cases which take a favourable turn, the patient becomes less benumbed and less indifferent, his sleep is quieter; appetite gradually returns. The bronchial catarrh grows better, the stool once more becomes normal; in short, the patient enters the stage of convalescence.

This is a short sketch of the course the illness usually takes.

Of the deviations and complaints accompanying Abdominal Typhus, the following are the most important details: —

The fever takes its course in strict accordance with the described anatomical changes in the intestines. It increases gradually during the first week, and at the end of that period it reaches its maximum of about 104°. It stays at that point during the second stage, gradually sinking during the third stage.

In lighter cases the second stage may be extraordinarily short.

If perforation of the intestines, heavier bleeding or general collapse should ensue, attention is directed thereto through sudden and considerable decrease in the temperature of the body. Pneumonia, inflammation of the inner ear and other accompanying complications also cause sudden access of fever.

Effect upon the digestive organs: The tongue is generally coated while the fever lasts; the lips are dry and chapped, and look brown from bleeding. If the patient is not carefully attended to during the extreme numbness, a fungus growth appears which forms a white coating over the tongue, the cavity of the mouth and the pharynx, and may extend into the oesophagus. Later on the tongue loses this coating and becomes red as before. Few symptoms are shown by the stomach, except occasional vomiting and lack of appetite. During convalescence there is great desire for food. The anatomical changes in the intestines have already been mentioned.

While obstruction prevails during the first week, the second week is characterized by diarrhoea of a pale and thin consistency.

When general improvement sets in, the stools gradually decrease in number, they grow more solid and finally reach the normal. The abdomen is not very sensitive to pressure and is usually intensely inflated with gas.

In the region of the right groin a cooing sound is often heard, caused by a liquid substance in the intestines, which can be felt under pressure of the finger.

Bleeding from the intestines is not infrequent and happens during the third week of the illness. It usually indicates a bad complication, since the result may be fatal. The stool assumes a tar-like appearance through the mixture of the coagulated blood with the faeces. Close attention must be given to minor hemorrhages, since they often herald others of a more intense nature.

In such extreme cases of serious complications, however, a cure has nevertheless been sometimes effected. They are occasionally followed by the immediate beginning of convalescence.

The perforation of the intestines, which is caused by an ulcer eating its way through the wall of the intestines, is much more dangerous. It happens most frequently during the third or the fourth week. The patient feels a sudden, most intense pain in the abdomen; he collapses rapidly, the cheeks become hollow, the nose pointed and cool. Vomiting follows, the pulse becomes weak and extremely rapid. The abdomen is enormously inflated and painful. In the severest cases death ensues, at latest, within two or three days, the cause being purulent and ichorous (or pus-laden) peritonitis.

Such extreme developments as these, however, are infrequent, since the illness, by timely attention according to the methods herein prescribed, will, as a rule, respond to the treatment and take a favourable turn.

Respiratory Organs: —

In the course of typhus, intense bleeding of the nose is not infrequent. In the severer cases this is a sign of decomposition of the blood, but in lighter cases it merely serves to alleviate the intense headache which is a feature of the case. The throat is liable to be affected; hoarseness and coughing occur; hardly any case of typhus catarrh. This sometimes extends into the air-passes without a more or less intense bronchial cells and causes catarrhal pneumonia, which — if not promptly treated according to the instructions herein detailed — may become extremely dangerous.

Organs of Circulations: —

With the exception of a strongly accelerated action, no change is noticeable in the heart. It may, however, suddenly become paralyzed and cease entirely, owing to the general weakness of the patient and the intensity of the fever. Weakness of the heart and possible cessation occur only during the climax or convalescence.

Nervous System: —

Disturbances of the nervous system are very frequent, hence the name "nervous fever."

Consciousness is, in nearly all cases, more or less benumbed, and at times completely lost. The patient is either lying absolutely indifferent, or he is delirious, cries, rages, attempts to jump out of bed and can only be subdued by the strongest efforts.

Patients lose control of urinary and faecal movements and require feeding.

These disturbances disappear as soon as convalescence sets in and consciousness returns.

As a rule the patient, on return to consciousness, knows nothing of what he has gone through, and has no reminiscences of the immediate past.

Sometimes cramps in the masticatory muscles have been observed, which explains the grinding of teeth apparent in some instances. Convulsions in the limbs and facial muscles sometimes appear, but most of these disturbances are of short duration.

Urinary and Sexual Organs: —

With high fever albumen appears in the urine. In some instances it may lead to inflammation of the kidneys, the symptoms of which may at times completely overshadow the symptoms of typhus. Fortunately this complication is very rare. Catarrh of the bladder occurs, because the patient retains the urine too long, while in a state of unconsciousness. Inflammation of the testicles has been observed with male patients, and pregnant women have miscarried or given birth prematurely.

Bones and Joints: —

Inflammation of the joints is infrequent and in a few cases only, inflammation of the periosteum has been observed.

Skin: —

At the beginning of the second week small rose-like spots of a light rose colour appear on the buttocks (roseola typhosa), which later on are also found on the upper legs, upper arms and back. They soon disappear, however, and leave no traces.

Pustular eczema is so rare in cases of typhus, that as a rule its appearance is taken to indicate that the disease is not a case of abdominal typhus. Frequently, however, urticaria, (nettle-rash) perspiration and other pustules are to be noticed.

The great variety of symptoms indicates that innumerable peculiarities may occur in the course of typhus. In some cases it is so light and indistinct (walking typhoid) that it is extremely difficult to diagnose it. In other cases pneumonia or unconsciousness, headache or stiff neck are indicated so overwhelmingly, that it is well-nigh impossible to recognize the underlying illness as typhus. In such cases one speaks of lung and brain typhus.

Recurrence: —

In about 10% of all cases recurrence is observed, mostly caused through mistakes in diet, leaving bed too soon, and excitement. Usually in such relapses the fever takes the same course as the original attack, but is much less intense. Although such secondary attacks are not very dangerous as a rule, great caution should be observed, especially in regard to diet, which must be followed in the strictest way until all danger has passed.

Complications and Subsequent Troubles: — are very frequent and a serious menace to life.

The most important are hemorrhage of the brain, meningitis, erysipelas, gangrene of the skin and bones, wasting of the muscles, fibrinous pneumonia; pericarditis, and frequently weakness of the heart with its consequences.

Purulent inflammation of the middle ear is one which deserves special attention.

Loss of hair is a frequent occurrence during convalescence, owing to the ill-nourished condition of the skin; this, however, is but a temporary feature soon succeeded by renewed growth.

The prognosis or forecast of typhus is not altogether bad, notwithstanding the gravity of its symptoms and the dangers of its course.

Statistics show that the mortality from typhus does not exceed 7% but each complication makes the result more uncertain and the outlook less hopeful. In the event of perforation of the intestines and severe internal hemorrhage supervening, the chances of saving life are slender.

D. Treatment.

The treatment of typhus requires, in the first place, a correct judgment of the physical condition of the patient in determining the fever treatment to be applied. Success in severe cases of typhus will only be secured by those who understand the correct methods of treating the skin. Robust patients, with reserve energy and resisting power, may receive the unrelaxing application of repeated whole packs or cool full baths. There is, however, a species of endurance, which may prove unable to endure the sustained and active force of these applications. In such cases milder applications and more frequent changes are recommended. Packs, interchanged with baths, clysters or enemas which subdue fever, alternated with ablutions, and similar methods.

Extremely stout and nervous patients must be treated with the greatest caution.

As typhus cases gradually develop, care must be exercised to prevent too violent treatment in case of serious complications. In fact the physician must not be guided by fixed rules, but must be able to individualize with prompt discretion.

During the severest stage the diet must be absolutely a fever diet, prescribed in Form II, while patients suffering from lighter attacks, and convalescents, may be permitted the milder fever diet, given in Form III.

Mental Condition. Great care and observation is necessary with regard to the patient's mental state. The observance of a quiet demeanour on the part of everyone about the sick room should help to keep the patient quiet and undisturbed and may serve to preserve his consciousness.

I have treated very severe cases of typhus, with extremely high fever, during which, however, consciousness remained. Inexorable strictness in this respect is often resented and misunderstood by those surrounding the patient until they realize the far-reaching importance of the orders by comparison with other cases.

Cold ablutions on the affected parts, air and water cushions, must be employed early enough to avert any danger of bed-sores.

This strict treatment of the patient — physically and mentally, will in most cases be sufficient to render his condition endurable; otherwise the struggle against the irritation of complications becomes intense, rendering it imperative, in the first degree, that the brain symptoms should be carefully watched.

Cold compresses on the head must be used in case such symptoms appear, but absolute undisturbed rest will conduce more than anything else to their infrequent occurrence.

Collapse must be contended against with light stimulating food (light bouillon of veal or chicken with a little condensed substance). Wine with alcohol might endanger the life of the patient. If the collapse is protracted, constituting a menace to life, the addition of cold water to the lukewarm bath and similar procedure may be tried, but only by a skilled expert.

Diarrhoea must be resisted by means of diet and clysters (enemas) with rice-water, if necessary; the enemas must be given *cautiously*. They are dangerous on account of possible violations and consequently rupture of the ulcerated intestines. These and other points, however, such as threatening paralysis etc., are entirely in the hands of the physician.

The contest against all the complications of typhus must be directed by absolutely skilled and experienced persons only, since in this disease particularly every mistake of any importance whatsoever, may cost the life of the patient.

Besides this specific form of typhus which commands general attention, the others are of merely theoretical interest. One, however, I wish to mention in passing; namely:

E. Relapsing Fever (Typhus Recurrens).

This also begins with chills and shivering, and a general tired feeling, and is immediately followed by high fever, up to a temperature of 104°. The skin is covered with excretory perspiration. The brain symptoms are lacking. The illness reaches its climax very quickly; but suddenly the patient feels much better, after extremely free perspiration. He continues remarkably well for about a week, when a new attack of the illness, a relapse, occurs. There are frequently from three to four relapses of this kind, which severely tax the strength of the patient.

The number and the intensity of these relapses determines the degree of the illness.

The treatment is regulated in accordance with the principles to be applied in abdominal typhus. The relapses may be averted or at any rate reduced to a great degree, by strict observance of the methods herein prescribed, especially in regard to diet.

F. Diet in Cases of Typhus.

Typhus abdominalis is a form of disease which requires the most careful dietetic treatment, since it combines high fever, which lasts for several weeks, with a severe ulcerous process in the small and large intestines.

Nutrition is seriously hampered by the long duration of the illness, usually considerable lack of appetite and the absolute necessity of nursing the ulcerous intestines in the most studiously careful way.

In cases which develop to the highest degree, it naturally follows that the patient wastes away to a great extent.

In the first place, all solid food must be strictly avoided. Too great stress cannot be laid on this point, since the patient, especially in lighter cases, frequently shows a strong desire for food—especially fruit.

Any lack of firmness and caution in this respect may have the most disastrous consequences. Many a patient suffering from typhus has lost his life or experienced a bad relapse and hemorrhages of the intestines through a mistake in diet, — through taking too much or unsuitable food.

The most critical period for the liability to hemorrhage, which in some cases is very profuse, is the third, and in lighter cases, the second week, when the crust of the intestinal ulcers begins to scale off.

The diet list, as in cases of typhus, consists of Form II, and milk; and it should be made a rule to confine it strictly to the most simple food, bouillon, mucilaginous soups, milk, undiluted or with tea, everything prepared with a little egg. Cream will sometimes agree with the patient.

The stools will indicate the digestion or otherwise of the milk. If there are many morsels of casein apparent in the same, the quantity of milk must be reduced and given in diluted form. The use of meat juice, liquid or frozen, and meat jelly, is quite permissible. Although neither of these preparations are very strong, they must be considered as important building-stones for the nourishment of the patient, and they offer a little variety, which is often most desirable.

Drinks. For drinking, usually fresh water is used, also bread and albumen water, especially Dechmann's Plasmogen, 15 grains in one pint of water, a mouthful from time to time alternating with Dechmann's Tonogen.

Great caution must be used in regard to fruit juices and lemonade on account of the danger of irritation of the intestines.

Carbonated and other mineral waters must be strictly avoided, since they only add to the usually prevailing meteorism, or gas in the abdominal cavity.

Albumen water, which is occasionally used in case of febrile disease and intestinal catarrh of children, is prepared by mixing the white of an egg and two to four spoonfuls of sugar in a tumbler of water. This is strained and cooled before being used. It is easily understood that by this we generate new life in the patient, so to speak, through the albumen, since it contains a large quantity of tissue building material, which in turn prevents catabolism or destruction of the organism, this as contrasted with the methods of the old regime which dooms the patient to certain death by opiates, — a course frequently resorted to by inexperienced practitioners.

If, by attention and care, the treatment has succeeded in strengthening the energy of the resisting organism to a certain degree during the fever, it becomes necessary in due course to regulate the desire for food, which sometimes grows and asserts itself in a rapid and energetic manner, while the fever is receding.

The cessation of fever by no means indicates that the ulcers are completely healed, and any mistake as to quantity and quality of food may cause a relapse. Liquid diet must, therefore, be given exclusively for at least, another eight days after the fever has ceased. After this, from week to week, gradually, the use of Form III, may be employed and thereafter more solid food, as given anon, under Form IV.

These cautions must be strictly heeded, especially in case of typhus recurrens.

If in the course of typhus severe complications, such as hemorrhage of the intestines or perforation thereof, should supervene, nourishment must immediately be reduced to a minimum. In such instances it is best to confine the diet to mucilaginous soup and to forbid everything else, as long as hemorrhages have not ceased, or the other dangerous peritonitic symptoms have not disappeared. Gradually, Form V and lastly, Form VI, may be followed.

Form IV. Diet of the lightest kind, containing meat, but only in scraped or shredded form. Noodle soup, rice soup.

Mashed boiled brains or sweetbread, or puree of white or red roasted meat, in soup.

Brains and sweetbread boiled.

Raw scraped meat (beef, ham, etc.)

Lean veal sausages, boiled.

Mashed potatoes prepared with milk.

Rice with bouillon or with milk.

Toasted rolls and toast.

Form V. Light diet, containing meat in more solid form.

Pigeon, chicken boiled.

Small fish, with little oil, such as brook or lake trout, boiled.

Scraped beefsteak, raw ham, boiled tongue.

As delicacies: small quantities of caviar, frogs' legs, oysters, sardelle softened in milk.

Potatoes mashed and salted, spinach, young peas mashed, cauliflower, asparagues tips, mashed chestnuts, mashed turnips, fruit sauces.

Groat or sago puddings.

Rolls, white bread.

Form VI. Somewhat heavier meat diet. (Gradually returning to ordinary food.)

Pigeon, chicken, young deer-meat, hare, everything roasted.

Beef tenderloin, tender roast beef, roast veal.

Boiled pike or carp.

Young turnips.

All dishes to be prepared with very little fat, butter to be used exclusively. All strong spices to be avoided. Regarding drinks to be taken with these forms of diet, as a rule good drinking water takes the first place. This is allowed under all circumstances. Still less irritating are weak decoctions of cereals, such as barley and rice water. Other light nutritive non-irritating drinks are bread water and albumen water.

Only natural waters, such as Vichy, Apollinaris with half milk or the like are to be used. Drinks containing fruit acid, like lemonade and fruit juices, are somewhat stimulating; however, in a general way, they may be given during fever, but not in typhus.

Of alcoholic drinks the best is light wine (bordeaux), first diluted and later in its natural state. As a rule it should not be used before Form IV has been followed and Form V commenced. Occasionally, mild white wine or well fermented beer, may be permitted. Coffee is absolutely forbidden during any of the foregoing forms of diet, but light teas with milk are allowed in most cases.

The main point in the different forms of diet as enumerated herein is to be found in the mechanical gradation of the substances in accordance with the progressive condition of the patient.

The diet in a certain individual case of the kind will not, however, always be necessarily identical with one or any of the foregoing forms, but must depend upon the individual condition.

In the first place, under each form there are easily discernible gradations, according to relative points of view which are all familiar to the physician and to which attention must be paid under similar circumstances. On the other hand, very often one of the items of a later form may be allowed while, in general, one of the previous forms is applied. Thus the transition from Form II to the first items of Form III is hardly perceptible.

Of course every form comprises all previous ones, so that each consecutive form affords a greater range than the last.

Occasionally other points than those I have mentioned may have to be taken into consideration. It is obviously impossible as the reader will observe, to formulate an absolutely uniform scheme applicable to every case.

Next to the description and quality of food, the quantity to be introduced into the stomach at one time, is a matter of the utmost vital importance.

DECH-MANNA-COMPOSITIONS.

(Only main compositions, specialities to Doctor's order.)

In all forms of Typhoid fever: **Neurogen**, **Plasmogen**, **Tonogen**, Eubiogen.

Physical: Partial Packs.

SO-CALLED "NEGATIVE CHILDREN'S DIS-EASE".

In strong contrast to the conditions of "positive" disease amongst children, due, as I have explained, to over-vitality and too rapid vibrations, we have to consider the opposite condition of Negative disease, comprising all physical disturbances wherein cold negative electrical forces and reduced vibrations produce unhealthy action of the mucous membranes, resulting in degeneration of the tissues known as Catarrh in various forms. Bronchitis, Grippe, Influenza and light catarrhal inflammation of the respective organs. One of the most serious in this chapter is summer-complaint (Cholera infantum). This disease, which causes the death of so many, is due to the bringing up of infants on artificial food instead of on the mother's breast. It is one of the negative diseases caused by diminished vitality. The disease is similar to Asiatic cholera. An extensive description of the same is given in Chapter XI A of my book, "Regeneration or Dare To Be Healthy." Frequent vomiting and diarrhoea, with rapid collapse of all vitality, and severe brain disturbances manifest themselves, and death frequently occurs after 36 hours. During hot weather bacterial germs impregnating the air, frequently enter the milk, and many children succumb to the disease at the same time, until wind and rain improve the general conditions. This is the explanation of the occasional epidemic appearance of Cholera Infantum—and its established cause.

Therapy.

Diet: The mother's breast or the breast of a healthy wet nurse is the very best remedy for this complaint, if applied at an early stage. If this is impossible, a gruel of barley, oats or mucilaginous rice-water, a decoction of salep (1 teaspoonful to 1 pint of water), or rice water (1 teaspoonful of crushed toasted rice to ½ pint water) are recommended. The missing nutritive substance is best supplied by calcareous earth (calcium carbonate), giving ¼ teaspoonful in a tablespoonful of sweetened water every 3 to 4 hours, for a day or two. It is the simplest, yet most wonderful remedy ever discovered. It is in cases like this that physiological chemistry celebrates its victory. Try it and you will be convinced. For more vigorous means the physician must be consulted, as he should be in any case of this kind, and that as quickly as possible.

Physical: Sponging the entire body of the child with lukewarm vinegar and water, using one-half vinegar and one-half water, may prove very successful. Warm packs around the abdomen and extending down to the soles of the feet, often prove very effective. The abdomen must be kept warm. The employment of coloured light for curative purposes has been already explained in the preceding pages. The use of *blue* curtains is, accordingly enjoined here on account of the invigorating influence of the more violent vibrations of *blue light* upon an organism suffering under the reduced vibration of a "negative disease."

The Contagious Character of Children's Diseases.

In strict adherence to the biological standpoint, it is recommended that a child be separated from the other children in the house as soon as it becomes ill, and if it is not convenient to send the other children away to be taken care of by friends, they must at least be excluded from the sick-chamber. *Each one of these diseases develops some sort of bacillus in its first appearance, and this leaves the body and may fall on receptive soil in the body of another child.* Since all the children in one family live in the same environment and receive practically the same nourishment, and are of the same parentage, the presumption prevails that each one of them is equally susceptible to the disease with which one of the children has been affected. It is, therefore, advisable to adopt preventive and protective measures with them all, by applying abdominal packs and giving them Dechmann's Plasmogen, which will strengthen the white corpuscles of the blood in their fight against possibly intruding bacilli; also Dechmann's Tonogen, in order to give the red corpuscles and the heart the power to endure the greater efforts which the demand for increased vitality will necessitate. The application of these measures will in many cases entirely prevent an impending attack of the disease, and if not, will at least make it easier to control.

The golden rule: Keep the head cool, the feet warm and the bowels open; that is the golden rule to be followed in the treatment of all children's diseases. All means that are applied must have but the one object, that of making the condition of the blood as good as possible, so that it will maintain a fluid form and circulate readily, richly supplied with all the necessary upbuilding substances. This, and not the use of anti-toxins, will guarantee a speedy return to normal conditions.

Diet: The importance of the diet in all of these diseases has been indicated on several occasions. Its application is treated extensively under the fever diet; exceptions to be determined by the physician.

Dech-manna-Compositions: The compositions to be used in case of children's diseases will, as indicated above, consist mainly of Plasmogen and Tonogen. Small doses of Eubiogen will be of great advantage in promoting the general condition of the patient. These three compositions should always be available in a family where there are children, as their application will prove very beneficial in any case, even before the arrival of the physician.

Physical: The correct application of ablutions of vinegar and water, of partial and other packs and various baths, must be left to the prescription of the physician, depending on the nature of the individual case, and the effect on the patient, with the exception of the abdominal pack. This should always be applied immediately: cold in positive, and warm in negative diseases.

THE TONSURE OF THE TONSILS.

Though not strictly within the scope of my intention in the present booklet, I feel that no treatise, however brief, which purports to be a free and candid expression of the ills that child-life is heir to, could afford to ignore the burning and much debated question of the tonsils and their significance, present and future, to the well-being of the child, or could deem the task accomplished without raising a warning and protesting voice on behalf of the helpless victims, whose recurrent name is legion, against the callous and persistent violation and destruction of the functions of vital organs, the only shadow of justification of which is, on the one hand, a fashionable popular delusion on the part of parents and, on the other, interested complacency on the part of their medical advisers, accentuated by a strong and dangerous tendency towards operation and empiric surgery generally.

This is a strong and sweeping indictment, perhaps. Let us therefore pause for a moment whilst we consult other sources of opinion for confirmation or refutal.

And, in the wide range of American and English criteria, what corroboration do we find? We find, as regards America, the venerable Professor Alexander H. Stevens, M.D., a member of the New York College of Physicians, writing as follows:

"The reason medicine has advanced so slowly is because physicians have studied the writings of their predecessors instead of nature."

From England the verdict comes to this effect:

Professor Evans, Fellow of the Royal College of Physicians and Surgeons, of London, says, in part:

"The Medical Practice of our day is, at the best, a most uncertain and unsatisfactory system: it has neither philosophy nor common sense to recommend it to confidence."

If such opinions prevail *within* the sacred, State-protected precincts of the profession, how long, revolted confidence exclaims—

how long before a credulous, deluded public awakens from its deep hypnotic trance.

Against Tonsil destruction three arguments stand:

(1) That the primal intention of Universal Mind — (sometimes termed the Soul of Being; the Spirit of All Good or, in simple reverence, "God") — was obviously no malign intention, but an intention for *good*, is an axiom which will be rationally accepted, I presume, as logically and conclusively assured.

(2) That the functions of the tonsils are, in the present state of medical knowledge, practically still unknown is the deliberate and final statement made within the past few years by one of the greatest reputed authorities on the subject.

(3) That the tonsil has some important mission to fulfill is clearly demonstrated by the fact of its frequent recrudescence, or rather, the natural renewal of the organ after surgical removal — a spontaneous physiological organic mutiny, as it were, supported by its lymphatic glandular dependents, against the reckless ignorance of medical practitioners and the perversity of the medico-cum-parental fashion of the day.

For the fact that it is a fashion, and nothing more, is unhappily fully established on ample and high authority within the medical prescriptive pale. And, in fact, even as "The Tonsure" or shaving of the crown, became by fashion and mendicity a feature of priesthood and monastic piety, so has the slaughter of the Tonsils come to be regarded by fashion and mendacity as a feature of childhood and medical expediency and ineptitude.

Professor John D. Mackenzie, M.D., of Baltimore, a distinguished leader of the advanced school of medical science, in the course of a brilliant and exhaustive treatise on the subject written as he says, reluctantly, in the interest of the public health and safety, quotes the deliberate opinion of an equally eminent medical friend to the effect that:

"Of all the surgical insanities within his recollection this onslaught on the tonsils was the worst — not excepting the operation on the appendix."

Dr. Mackenzie then proceeds to show how abysmal has been the ignorance of the functions of these organs from the earliest times, (including a distinguished English medical luminary who went to far as to say: "were I attempting the artificial construction of a man I would leave out the tonsils,") adding that the tonsil was regarded as a useless appendage and "like its little neighbour, the uvula, was sacrificed on every possible pretext or when the surgeon did not know what else to do."

"Never," he says, "in the history of medicine has the lust for operation on the tonsils been as passionate as it is at the present time. It is not simply a surgical thirst, it is a mania, a madness, an obsession. It has infected not only the general profession, but also the laity." In proof of this he adds: "A leading laryngologist in one of the largest cities came to me with the humiliating confession that although holding views hostile to such operations he had been forced to perform tonsillectomy in every case in order to satisfy the popular craze and to save his practice from destruction." He cites an instance in which a mother brought her little six-year-old daughter to him, "to know whether her tonsils ought to come out;"—and in answer to the assurance: "your baby is perfectly well, why do you want her tonsils out?" the fond mother's reply was: "Because she sometimes wets the bed!"

Recent universal inspection of the throats of school children has revealed the fact that nearly all children at some time of life have more or less enlarged tonsils. And the reports maintain that this, for the most part, is harmless if not actually physiologic—natural—and that their removal in these cases is not only unnecessary but injurious to the proper development of the child.

Nevertheless, the reports of the special hospitals for diseases of the nose and throat show to what an appalling extent this destructive operation is perpetrated throughout the land.

"Much wild and incontinent talk," Dr. Mackenzie continues, "for which their teachers are sometimes largely to blame, has poisoned the minds of the younger generation of operators and thrown the public into hysteria. They are told that with the disappearance of the tonsils in man, certain diseases will cease to exist and parents nowadays bring their perfectly sound children for tonsil removal in order to head off these affections. Summing up the writer demonstrates that the functions of the tonsils are, at present unknown and that until known nothing authoritative can be said definitely on the subject, whether they be portals for the entrance of disease or the exit for the very purpose of germs of infection; common sense must decide;—whether they protect the organism from danger or invite the presence of disease."

I, for my own part, am of Dr. Mackenzie's opinion: that there is an endless flow of lymph from their interior to the free surface, which unchecked, *prevents the entrance of germs from the surface and washes out impurities from within*. That in any case, one of the functions undoubtedly is the production of leucocytes or protective white blood corpuscles and that the tonsil is not, as generally understood, a lymphatic gland; that the general ignorance of this fact has led to the useless sacrifice of thousands of tonsils, on the fallacious assumption that their functional activities may be vicariously undertaken by other lymphatic glands; and finally, that the physiologic integrity of the tonsil is of the utmost importance in infant and child life.

The consensus of advanced scientific opinion is now to the effect that the activity of the tonsils as possible accessories of disease has been vastly exaggerated, that like the thousand and one successive misleading theories which in turn, from time to time, have seized upon the imagination and obsessed the minds of the medical fraternity for brief and passing periods, this pernicious craze too, has about run its course. The causes from which this peculiar lust for operation emanates would be perhaps a difficult psychological puzzle to determine; the malign impulse, as regards some special function, seems to spring, as it were, by intuition, unbidden into being from the illusive depths of some perverted intellect, to rage for a while through the medical world with a death roll deadly as the plague and as suddenly to pass into desuetude and disappear behind the impregnable ramparts of "prescriptive right" and "privilege"—terms which in plain parlance mean to the masses in cold actual fact, the absolute negation of all right—the domination of arbitrary, irresponsible and State protected wrong.

Between facts and fables, the evidence with regard to the tonsils and their functions seems to establish the conclusion that they have been wrongfully and foolishly held responsible for "an iliad of ills." The region of the nose and mouth is obviously the happy hunting-ground of myriads of pathogenic bacteria. It is likewise continually the scene of innumerable surgical operations, performed necessarily without antiseptic precautions, thus extending the area of possible infection indefinitely to the entire upper air tract which medical incompetence so often fails to explore. And indeed, as Dr. Macken-zie freely remarks: "Of far graver, far-reaching and deeper signifi-cance are cases of infection in which life has doubtless been sacri-ficed by clinging to the lazy and stupefying delusion that the tonsil is the sole portal of poisoning."

The mere size of the tonsil, it is shown, is no indication for re-moval except it be large enough or diseased enough to interfere with respiration, speech or deglutition—that is, swallowing; in which case only a sufficient portion should be taken away, and that without delay. The tonsil may be greatly enlarged or buried deeply in the palatine arcade and yet not interfere with the well-being of the individual. Such tonsils are the special prey of the tonsillecto-mist. If they are not interrupting function they are best left alone. Moreover, it occasionally happens that the resurrection of a "buried" tonsil is followed shortly by the *burial of the patient.*

The practical illuminating lesson to be gleamed is this: That if in infancy and childhood, we pay more attention to the neglected na-sal cavities and to the hygiene of the mouth and teeth, we will have less tonsil disease and fewer tonsil operations.

"The partial enucleation of the tonsil," the writer asserts, "with even the removal of its capsule if desired, is complete enough for all necessary purposes and practically free from danger; moreover, it produces equal or better results than complete enucleation with its many accidents and complications, to say nothing of its long roll of *unrecorded death.*"

Another point: From the professional vocalist's point of view. The tonsils are phonatory or vocal organs and play an important part in the mechanism of speech and song. They influence the surrounding muscles and modify the resonance of the mouth. Enlarged by disease, they may cripple these functions and if so, their removal may increase the compass of the voice by one or more octaves; but it is a capital operation and a dangerous one in which a fatal result is by no means a remote possibility.

The object of this interesting paper, it is pointed out, is not to assail operation for definite and legitimate cause, but to warn against the "busy internist"—the hospital surgeon—too busy for careful differential diagnosis—and his "accommodating tonsillectomist" who is "in the business for revenue only." But the onus for the existing deplorable state of affairs he lays frankly upon the shoulders of the teachers and insists that the cure of the evil is largely educational. "When," says he, "*pre-eminent authority proclaims in lecture and text book as indisputable truth the relationship between a host of diseases and the tonsils of the child and advises the removal of the glands as a routine method of procedure, what can we expect of the student whose mind is thus poisoned at the very fountainhead of his medical education by ephemeral theory that masquerades so cheerily in the garb of indestructible fact*?" "How," he exclaims, "are we to offset the irresponsibility of the responsible?" But we hear on all sides—"Look at the results." Results? Here is a partial list from the practice—not of the ignorant, but of the most experienced and skilled: Death from hemorrhage and shock, development of latent tuberculosis, laceration and other serious injuries of the palate and pharyngeal muscles, great contraction of the parts, removal of one barrier of infection, severe infection of wound, septicemia, or bacterial infection, troublesome cicatrices, suppurative otitis media and other ear affections, troubles of voice and vision, ruin of singing voice, emphysemia, or destruction of the tissues, septic infarct,—infected arterial obstruction, pneumonia, increased susceptibility to throat disease, pharyngeal quinsy and last, but not least tonsillitis!

The trenchant and tragic article concludes with the expression of the hope that the day is not far distant when not only the profession but the public shall demand that this senseless slaughter be stopped. "Is not this day of medical and moral preaching and uplifting," it is asked, "a fitting one in which to lift the public out of the atmosphere into which it has been drugged, and as to the reckless tonsillectomist, a proper time to apply the remedy of the *referendum* and *recall*. It has come to a point when it is not only a burning question to the profession, but also to the public. This senseless, ruthless destruction of the tonsil is often so far reaching and enduring in its evil results that it is becoming each day a greater menace to the public good."

> Such is the wisdom of these world-wide sages,
> They wildly yearn to learn its innermost
> And break the organ's wondrous works with sledges—
> Though music, its sweet soul, for aye is lost;
> That they have reached the goal, such is their dreaming,
> When tissues, nerves, and veins reveal their knife—
> When in the very core their steel is gleaming—
> But, one thing they forget—*and that is life*!

This matter of the functions of the tonsils is fully dealt with in my greater work "Regeneration or Dare to be Healthy"—Chapters VII. and VIII., in which I show on the best authority that *the tonsils have a great mission to fulfill*—so great indeed that their treatment according to the present methods of the medical faculty can, in my estimation, only be stigmatized as the equivalent of a crime.

It is the conclusion arrived at scientifically by the greatest authorities that the Tonsils secrete a very potent anti-toxic fluid which is excreted whenever dangerous pathogenic bacilli attempt to enter the pharynx or larynx, constituting in fact the ever watchful sentinels of the oral and nasal portals through which an entrance into the human organism might be surprised by its ever active surreptitious enemies—the bacteria of infection and disease.

PRE-NATAL CARE.

It would be improper to close this section, touching child-life, without some special reference to pre-natal care. It has been well said by eminent authorities that a child's *"education should begin long before its birth."* This to many may seem mysterious or even foolish, according to their advancement on the plane of knowledge. But America has long ago awakened to the truth of it, and pre-natal clinics have been established on a large scale—notably in New York—for the scientific supervision and comfort of expectant mothers who may need it. The natural right of every child to be born in health and happiness, is at length recognized.

Human magnetism, or nerve force, is beginning to be understood and utilized as a great vital, health-compelling, harmonizing factor of vast significance to the future of the race.

The real and practical alliance between the physical and the psychic—between body and mind—is better realized; as for instance: You may be seized with *an idea*, or a passion, and it disturbs your *health of body*; you may take indigestible food, or suffer injury or fatigue, and it disturbs your *health of mind.*

But beyond and behind all else are all those seemingly occult and sinister, pre-natal influences centered in hereditary and kindred considerations which are still more significant and difficult to locate and overcome.

These problems have been thought out and solved long before the dawn of the present social awakening and the conclusions have been tabulated in the closest detail from the first moment of embryonic life, faithfully defining the paths that inevitably lead to the desired goal of Hygienic Birth, of Physical Perfection and the Mental State termed Happiness, in Infancy.

All these things will be found minutely focussed in picturesque relief, in my previous work entitled: "Within the Bud."

ENDEMIC AND EPIDEMIC DISEASE.

Among the most deadly menaces that beset human life upon this planet are those forms of disease classed under the head of so-called Endemic and Epidemic disease and including in its baleful limits Yellow fever, Cholera, Pellagra—otherwise known as Hook-worm, Plague and so-called Spanish Influenza.

Based upon Physiological Chemistry and explained from the Biological standpoint, the explanation of these covers a wide scientific area and geographically treated embraces the globe.

The various problems of their cause and prevention have exercised the mind of science and research to an enormous degree and heavy premiums have been placed upon their solution, with more or less success and much expenditure has been incurred in the examination of local conditions.

As far as this Continent is concerned, perhaps the most troublesome has been Climatic Fever which varies greatly in form and intensity according to temperature and location.

"Yellow Fever," as it is named, has swept some Southern localities from time to time, but Science, Sanitation and Hygiene have curbed its virulence and spread, as in the case of outbreaks of epidemics such as small-pox—for the control of which, by the way, the advocates of the vile and pernicious practice of vaccination, fraudulently claim the credit, even in these advancing times, when the wiles of self interest are disclosed, the worship of the "Putrid Calf" exposed and the days of the vaccine vendor numbered.

Yellow Fever occurs on the Coast of tropical countries and, as a rule, is fatal, after a rapid development of from 3 to 7 days.

The explanation of the cause of the disease is comparatively simple: The air on the hot coast lands is highly charged with evaporated water. Heat and humidity have the effect of diverting from the human organism the electricity which, as already shown, constitutes its vital cohesion and the same influences likewise reduce the oxygen in the atmosphere. These are the two primary causes of Yellow Fever.

Pellagra (hook-worm or Lombardy Leprosy) is, according to the tenets of the Regular School, an endemic skin and spinal disease of Southern Europe. It is said to be due to eating damaged corn but dependent also upon bad hygienic conditions, poor food and exposure to the sun. Its salient features are weakness, debility, digestive disturbance, spinal pain, convulsions, melancholia and idiocy.

More recent investigation has judged it to be a deficiency disease, due to low and unvaried diet and consequent failure of metabolism.

In every case these climatic disease forms are caused by a combination of hot air, lacking oxygen, and evaporated water, including Cholera which also varies in intensity according to heat conditions.

Cholera and Plague originate on the coast of Bengal, India, where conditions are bad enough of themselves without the apology of the illusive bacillus as a causative agent.

That Cholera is contagious cannot be doubted and it is no superstition that fear predisposes thereto. For all emotions consume electrical power in the body and thus break down its power of resistance.

Infantile paralysis, Typhoid-fever, Small-pox, etc., are dealt with elsewhere and therefore need no mention here.

It is impossible to deal adequately with so wide a subject within the narrow limits at my disposal; but the full details and environment of each, together with the respective methods of treatment will be found in detail in the parent work "Regeneration or Dare to be Healthy."

THE SPANISH INFLUENZA.

In any attempt to unravel the tangled skein of cause and circumstance which surrounds the subject of the world-sweeping pandemic which masquerades under the misleading title of the "Spanish Influenza," the first and most important initial step must be a keen and careful sifting of the facts and forces, natural and artificial, which control or dominate the situation.

The debatable questions appear to be chiefly the following:

(1) The fundamental causes that underlie the great-epidemics or pandemics that the world experiences from time to time—the present one in particular.

(2) The fact or fallacy of the germ as a causative factor or merely an effect or product of disease conditions.

(3) The alternative course, origin and medium of transmission and finally

(4) The soundness and efficiency or otherwise of the preventive and curative measures with which the combined intelligence of the Medical Faculty has risen to the dire emergency of the moment for the protection of the people who have relied so confidently, as by law compelled, upon the standard of their acumen and official aid as competent guardians of public safety.

The findings, as to the first question, are to the effect that it appears, from the earliest recorded annals of disease, that epidemics corresponding to the present outbreak have occurred at irregular periods all up the centuries under names and conditions peculiar to the times, and following usually in the wake of some great social cataclysm, strain or upheaval, the result of wars, persecutions, famines and distress—causes which clearly illustrate the close reactive connection between the mental and physical action of disease.

The great pandemics seem to have originated largely in the Orient—the region of vast congested populations and racial struggles and starvation—the advent of their apparent influence upon the western world depending chiefly upon the rate of commercial or popular intercourse, the movements of armies or the ingress or egress of peoples. The logical establishment of direct proof of the connection between these visitations and local epidemics in distant lands is a problem as yet unsolved. The weight of evidence, at first sight, would seem to lie rather in the other direction—to indicate that such epidemics are the direct outcome of existing local conditions, mental and physical.

For example: At the end of that strenuous period in England's history, between the reign of the first Charles and the fall of the Commonwealth, an epidemic broke out which, as the historian tells us, converted the country into "one vast hospital." The malady—which by the way was fatal to Cromwell—the Lord Protector himself—was then termed "the ague." The term "Influenza" was first given to the epidemic of 1743 in accordance with the Italianizing fashion of the day, but was eventually superseded by the French expression "La Grippe," usually held to represent a more modified form of the disease which appears to vary in intensity and virulence according lo its provocation and derivation.

The old school hypothesis and the deductions therefrom would seem therefore, to be this: That a super-malignant contagium imported from some foreign source falls upon organisms predisposed to infection by mental stress or physical privation and over-strain or both combined; and the contagion thus generated through the medium of some unsuspected "carrier" seizes upon and sweeps through that portion of the community so predisposed, in the form of a great, general epidemic with a maximum of mortality. At later intervals the same repeats itself with less violence and reduced mortality, because a great proportion,—representing the sufferers in the original epidemic,—being now thereby immune, the onus falls upon that section of the younger generation unprotected by individual resistant force who consequently become the chief sufferers—as in the case of the present epidemic, the pandemic form of which is obviously due to the fact that equal conditions of unrest, privation and distress prevail universally throughout the entire nerve plains of the Planet.

The first recorded outbreak in America occurred in the year 1647, followed by a second in 1655 and again in 1789 and 1807. In these the mortality appears to have been confined, after the first outbreak, to a few mere modest thousands whereas in the present visitation a conservative estimate places the figures of the horrible world-holocaust at no less a sum than 18 *million lives* in all. [D] The ravages in America have been appalling including many of the medical profession.

We pass on then to the second item — the question of the germ.

The illusive germ has come to be regarded by the layman with reserve — nay more — with suspicion. The part of the bacteriologist has been somewhat overdone. The conditions of popular credence are not what they were. A great change has awakened the masses of the people and a new intelligence is born which now discerns that disease is one great Unity just as the body is one inseparable interdependent whole — that *the cause of disease is in the blood* and dependent upon its nourishment and moreover, that the *physical forces of the body can be exhausted as much by mental strain, — causing the too rapid burning up of nerve fat (lecithin), — as by excessive physical exertion.* For example. Mental disturbance — grief, worry, excitement — produce immediate physical effect in headache, palpitations and the like. Physical exhaustion — privation, hunger and over-work — on the other hand produce mental depression and collapse. The inevitable law of compensation rules.

Thus the germ, bacillus, or microbe, as a direct *cause* of disease is an exploded fallacy. They are now recognized as the *result* of disease — *not the cause*: releasing irritants perhaps and possibly carriers or transmitting mediums to other diseased or predisposed organisms.

It follows accordingly that Sero-Therapy or Inoculation with specific serums derived from such germs, as a preventative of disease is simply a pernicious farce; "pernicious," since the introduction of such poisons by inocculation into the blood constitutes in itself a serious menace to life and health.

This has never been more clearly demonstrated than in the present singularly futile efforts of the Regular Medical Faculty to stay the on-rush of the Influenza Epidemic or to save or safeguard its victims — a fact which compels the people in their thousands to turn to the less pretentious but more successful members of the eclectic or Irregular schools among whom both help and healing may be found.

And this is the history of the Influenza germ:

The bacterial criminal was located. We know it, for the discovery was officially proclaimed and vouched for by the press with all due pomp and circumstance. True, it was "so minute as to be *invisible to the most powerful microscope;*" — but it was sensed by science, none the less, and handed over captive, for "culture" to the *manufacturing chemist.* Inoculation followed freely — the people in their thousands and our gallant troops alike submitted to the mandate of the powers that be — the soldiers voiceless and under penalty.

America breathless, awaited the result. There was none.

Finally scare-heads in the Press astonished the land. They were these: *"Medical World is Baffled by the 'Flu'."* — *"Exhaustive Experiments Leave Doctors Mystified."* — *"Every Test a Failure."* — *"Explosion of Accepted Theories Causes Science to Grope for Light."*

It appears that, through the heroism of a *hundred* of our naval men who volunteered for the purpose at the risk of life, the Medical Authorities in desperation were enabled to try every possible method of infection with the alleged Influenza Germs, our boys submitting to inoculation and even to the repulsive ordeal of introduction into the nose and throat of diseased mucous from and close contact with coughing and spitting bed patients in the severest forms of the disease. The experiments were made simultaneously at San Francisco and Boston under the direction of Surgeons McCoy and Goldberger of the U.S. Health Department and the Naval Authorities.

The astounding negative result as indicated by the press, was described as "The Sensation of the day," for the fact was revealed that *Not one, of the hundred who underwent these drastic and determined tests, developed any symptoms of Influenza.* This picture of failure was surmounted by the summing up of the situation on the part of the highest Medical Authority; to this effect:

"These new experiments in the transmission of Influenza," said Surgeon General Blue, "show how difficult is the Influenza Problem."

The result points clearly to a state of natural immunity enjoyed by those who, like these men of the Naval Service, lead an hygienic, contented well regulated life with the simple accessories of good and sufficient food, fresh air and regular exercise.

The same principle has been recently demonstrated in England in the same connection by the annual report of one of the great public schools celebrated for hygienic methods, where amongst a total of 800 students not a single case of influenza appeared — although no preventive measures were employed beyond the simple rules of health and cleanliness.

Finally, as regards serums and specifics, the judgment of Dr. Karl F. Meyer, of the Hooper Institute of Medical Research of the University of California, may be accepted as focusing the consensus of unbiased opinion on the subject. It was as follows: "Serums have not yet been introduced which produce immunity from Spanish Influenza. The serums now employed are of no use whatsoever. You have no idea how really and truly helpless we are. As an example, take the advice given us by the Public Health Department when we asked what should be done if the epidemic struck West. They said: '*Organise your hospitals and undertakers.*'" In the same statement Dr. Meyer declared that the Medical fraternity *is in total darkness as to the cause and nature of the epidemic.*

Of other preventive measures resorted to — Masks, Quarantine and the veto upon public gatherings — proved equally mistaken and futile. Masks of a texture calculated to baffle the most determined attempts of the minute invisible homicide were made compulsory, and in the great cities masquerading millions became a constant feature of the streets, until an idea of the danger of masks, *as microbe preservers and carriers*, dawned upon the official mind. Thus, beyond fostering fear and depression amongst the citizens nothing was achieved in the direction desired, but rather the reverse; since it is now very generally recognized that such mental conditions with their consequently lowered vitality are a common prelude to disease.

At the annual meeting of the American Public Health Association in Chicago, following a two days' discussion of preventive measures against Influenza and Pneumonia, Dr. Chas. J. Hastings, president of the organization said: "A tremendous amount of damage is done by interfering with nature, when nature would have done better had she been left alone. We have very little power over pneumonia. I am convinced that as many patients have been *killed* by physicians as have been *cured*."

The talented "Health" editor of the Los Angeles Times, commenting upon these matters, writes: "The handling of this epidemic by 'health boards' and doctors who have been running around like wet chickens—their eyes, however, fastened on the feed box—has furnished another striking evidence of the futility of what is misnamed 'Medical Science.'"

All this carries one back 50 years to the memory of Sir John Forbes, Court Physician to the late Queen Victoria of England, and the eminent Editor of the British and Foreign Medical Review, who thus tersely recorded the scientific conclusions arrived at in the course of his long, professional experience, in connection with drugs, drug medication and allopathy, under the title of "Why we should not be poisoned because we are sick:" "Firstly,—that in a large proportion of cases treated by allopathic physicians, the disease is cured by nature and not by them. Secondly,—that in not a small proportion, the disease is cured by nature in spite of them. Thirdly,—that consequently, in a considerable proportion of diseases it would fare as well or better with patients if all remedies, especially drugs, were abandoned;" and he emphatically adds: "Things have come to such a pass that they must either mend or end." This, be it remembered, was in 1868,—50 years ago—and such frankness would not have been tolerated from other than "Sir John"—for, as was said by an inspired American: "He who dares to see a truth not recognized in creed must die the death." And now indeed is revealed the wisdom of Shakespeare when he said: "Ignorance is the Curse of God;" or of Bolinbroke's bitter assertion: "Plain truth will influence half a score men at most in a nation or an age, while *mystery will lead millions by the nose*."

I am not prepared to endorse the cynical saying of Voltaire: "Regimen is superior to medicine—especially as from time immemorial out of every hundred physicians ninety-eight are charlatans." But this much is certain, that they have found the needs of nature too laborious — the pathway of their leader — the Great Hippocrates — of Galen, Sydenham, Boerhaave, too tame, and have listened to the lure of Paracelsus, and adopted, with its high pontificial manner and medication, the more luxurious empiricism of the medicasters of five centuries ago.

But the time has come when the reign of bigotry, drugs and mystery must have an end — the chartered lien on human life must cease and the antique secret consistories so long omnipotent, must be brought to the enlightened level of the day.

We have come to the parting of the ways, where it becomes the bounden duty of every earnest, fair-minded physician to cast off the manacles of professional caste and secret obligation and to advance with open mind across the wholesome confines of eternal truth. This as much in their own interest as in that of their patients. For there is disaffection in the once solid phalanx, and we find strictures such as these in the standard works of the profession: "It cannot be denied that practitioners in medicine stand too low in the scale of public estimation and, something is rotten in the State of Denmark."

A series of articles appearing recently, in the English Review, from the daring and masterly pen of George Bernard Shaw, deals with the subject with an ungloved hand, taking as opportunity a vitriolic controversy recently raging between exalted lights of the medical profession in London, which raises abruptly the long-drawn curtain of mystery and exposes the secret skeleton to the view of a wondering world. Speaking of the absolute, autocratic powers of the medical monopoly and the superstitious, hopeless complacency of the public, the writer says: "The assumption is that the 'registered doctor' or surgeon knows everything that is known, and can do everything that is to be done. This means that the dogmas of omniscience, omnipotence and infallibility, and something very like the theory of the apostolic succession and kingship by anointment, have recovered in medicine the grip they have lost in theology and politics. This would not matter if the 'legally qualified doctor' was a *completely qualified healer*: but this is not the case; far from it. Dissatisfaction with the orthodox methods and technique is so widespread that the supply of technically qualified *unregistered* practitioners is insufficient for the demand.... The reputation of the unregistered specialist is usually well founded. *He must deliver the goods.* He cannot live by the faith of his patients in a string of letters after his name."

From all sides the same dissatisfaction is told showing that, with the sick and simple majority, what is termed "the attractive bed-side manner" of the polished practitioner has vastly out-weighed — in the past — the more vital advantage of superior skill on the part of practitioners of the drugless and natural systems which are winning their way to favour, in spite of the organized opposition of the orthodox profession and the powerful "vested interests" of the medicine-men.

To return to the subject proper: The summing up as to the efficacy of inoculation, drugs, serums and specifics for Influenza may best be found in the supplements to the U.S. Public Health reports, and vouched for by Surgeon-General Rupert Blue and the Government experts:

"Since we are uncertain of the primary cause of Influenza, no form of inoculation can be guaranteed to protect against the disease itself." "No drug has as yet been proved to have any specific influence as a *preventive* of influenza.

"No drug has as yet been proved to have any specific *curative* effect on influenza — though many are useful in guiding its course and mitigating *is symptoms.*

"In the uncertainty of our present knowledge considerable hesitation must be felt in advising vaccine treatment as a curative measure.

"The chief dangers of influenza lie in its complications, and it is probable that much may be done to mitigate the severity of the affection and to diminish its mortality *by raising the resistance of the body...."*

It is not my purpose in adducing these startling facts to impugn the Allopathic system or to disparage the elder branch of the Profession of Healing. They are simply assembled for the purpose of proving a case in favour of the newer or Hygieo-Dietetic System.

But here in consecutive order of testimony is a truly terrible denouncement—the testimony, as it were, of two hemispheres of the terrestrial globe proclaiming the positive failure of the section of science upon which, for very existence, their inhabitants have been accustomed to rely!

Now Health and Disease are dependent upon degrees of positive and negative vibrations, as is every form of life in the great Cosmic Unity of the Universe. Both are tones with endless modulation, but the integral fact, in either case, *is one*. Disease, then, is a Unit—a degenerate function of the blood—and, such being the case, the failure of any curative principle or system aspiring to remedy that degenerate functioning, in any degree, is a failure of that principle or system as a whole.

The sensational admission, therefore, of the chiefs of the Profession in America and England, as herein cited, amounts in plain language to the tacit admission that drugs and serums are powerless to produce any "preventive influence" or any "curative" effect upon Influenza, (or as it rationally and logically follows, upon any other disease) although, as openly stated in this official proclamation, they may influence the "symptoms."

But, finally—And here is the supreme announcement, wherein at length the Truth comes out triumphant—"The severity of the disease may be mitigated and its mortality diminished *by raising the resistance of the body.*"

This in one single sentence is the sum total of the teachings of the eclectic, independent and legally debarred and officially unrecognized Physiologico-Chemical, Hygieo-Dietetic School of Natural Science which I have the honor to represent.

The true teaching of Hippocrates, surnamed "The Father of Medicine"—the ostensible leader, for all time, of the "regular school" of Medicine was comprised in one phrase: the *Vis Medicatrix Naturae*—The Healing Power of Nature.

The teaching of our New, Independent School is identically the same—plus the physiologico-chemical discoveries of the intervening centuries. They are plain and natural precepts, surrounded by no fearsome atmosphere of mystery. They are to this effect:

415

That the human organism, together with all its interdependent parts, organs and functions, is an inseparable whole—a Unit—subject absolutely to Natural Laws. As said St. Paul: "And whether one member suffer, all the members suffer with it." (Cor. 12-26.)

That disease, therefore, is likewise a unit with a diversity of manifestations which, like all conflicting elements, develop in the individual organism along the lines of least resistance, according to the weakness—hereditary or acquired—of the individual. This we term predisposition.

The cause of predisposition to disease, centres absolutely and entirely in the blood, causing obstructions to normal circulation, the obstructing materials being poisons and impurities, either hereditary or acquired through malnutrition or the introduction of unassimilable matter into the system in the form of improper food, drugs, medicines or vaccines which remain as poisons in the blood.

Disease is the remedial effort of Nature to throw off such obstructions—a process of purification and regeneration—and its symptoms should be assisted and regulated rather than resisted and suppressed.

"Doctors prescribe—but only Nature cures," is an ancient axiom, but it faithfully represents the "*vis medicatrix naturae.*"

The question has recently been publicly propounded "Is sickness criminal?" Very certainly, disease is the outcome of personal neglect, in past or present; but the nature of the question is a sign significant that the laity are awakening to the truth that the healing power of nature rests wholly in the generation and conservation of latent reserve energy.

As regards the influenza controversy the Official verdict is, as we have seen, that the Regular Medical Profession as a whole, has failed in its endeavor to fathom the mystery and is at present "*really and truly helpless.*" Let us therefore, seek the cause of this disastrous failure and strive to solve the problem along other lines.

If so poor be the harvest, what of the soil? is the natural enquiry. And it must be generally admitted that this spectacular failure lies in the superficial teaching of the medical schools—its search for causes in the mature, and "specialized," anatomical organs in place of the fundamental physiological, chemical and embryonic causes from which, in their appointed order those various organs are evolved;—first the brain and nervous system, afterwards the tissues and the bones. Thus, unversed in the deeper phases of causation, men are hurried unprepared into ranks of a noble profession to struggle as best they may, through lack of deeper knowledge, with the serious symptoms of disease—at first by rote but later, are tempted to tamper empirically with its issues.

It has been said by a great scientific authority that, in order to thoroughly comprehend and cure any form of disease it is necessary, in the first place, to mentally map out and visualize the course of its growth and to follow it backward, step by step, to its source before it is possible to formulate curative treatment adapted to its cause and phases.

To commence then at the initial stage, let us bring upon the scene one of the greatest chemists of the age: Justus von Liebig, the discoverer of "The Law of the Minimum," which is this: That of the sixteen known constituents of the blood essential to the healthy growth and maintenance of the organs and tissues of the body, the absence of any proportional ingredient, however small, will cause degeneration in the organism and interfere with the proper functioning of one or more of the activities concerned.

Upon this Law is based the attested, dominant fact that all our mental and physical activities—powers of thinking, feeling, motion and every action, including the reproduction of species are equally dependent upon our blood—and our blood, in turn, depends upon proper nutrition. The ancient aphorism: "Man is as man eats," is therefore true in theory and in fact.

Human diet and human life being thus closely allied, it becomes a consideration of the first magnitude to see that all food contains in well balanced degree a correct proportion of the sixteen essentials: carbon, oxygen, hydrogen, nitrogen, iron, sulphur, phosphorus, chlorine, potassium, sodium, magnesium, calcium, manganese, fluorine, silicon and iodine.

Amongst the chemical salts of such scientific nutrition may, or may not, be found the famous "Vitamines," long sought of science; but what they certainly do supply is the electro-magnetic energy, the impulse of growth and vital function, the secret of bactericide blood and its power of circulation.

It is the magnetic iron in the blood which promotes nerve function in both the brain and the intestinal tract, producing on the one hand intellectual activity and on the other, breathing digestion and excretion. Similar causal action in corelation to the integral elements of food prevails throughout the organs of the body, demonstrating the vital importance of the quality of our daily food for the renewal of tissue and the maintenance of healthy metabolism.

In an attempt to define the *primary cause of Influenza*, Prof. Kuhnemann, a well known authority on practical and differential diagnosis, gives a minute description of its various *symptoms*, terminating with a weak suggestion that the already discredited bacillus *may be regarded as the cause.*

This is, in detail, as follows: "Fever is always present," Prof. Kuhnemann says, "but not of any certain type. At times, after short periods of Apyrexie there is a rise in temperature sometimes swelling of the spleen. There is no characteristic change in the urine; sometimes Albuminuria. There is an inclination to perspire freely; consequently Miliaria is often present; also Herpes, less frequently other Exanthema, Petechien. The mucous membranes are inclined to hemorrhage (Epistaxis, Hematemesis, Menorrhagia, Abortion).

"Complications and after effects:

(1) Of the respiratory system:—Croupose and Bronchopneumonia of atypical progress (atypical fever of protracted course, relatively strong Dyspnoe, Cyanosis, feeble pulse) and high mortality; after effects serous or mattery Pleuritis, Lung abscesses, Phthisis.

(2) Of the circulatory system:—Myocarditis, Endocarditis, Thrombosis.

(3) Of the digestive tract:—Chronic stomach and intestinal catarrh, Dyspepsia.

(4) Of the nervous system:—Any form of Neuralgia, Paralysis, Neuritis, Psychosis, etc.

(5) Of the sense organs:—Otitis media; Nephritis and Muscular Rheumatism are also observed. Influenza aggravates any case of sickness, especially lung trouble."

All this seems to constitute a very formidable and perplexing indictment, sparkling with learning and bristling with difficulties. But when these mellifluous mysticisms are once translated into "the vulgar tongue" they prove to be, strange to say, easily within the comprehension of the ordinary layman.

For instance, "Apyrexie" means Free from fever; Albuminuria—Albumen present; Miliaria—an acute inflammation of the sweat-glands (Abnormal sweating); Herpes—an inflammatory skin disease characterized by the formation of small vesicles in clusters (Fever rash); Exanthema—Skin eruption; Petechien—Spots; Epistaxis—Nose-bleeding; Hematemesis—vomiting blood; Menorrhagia—Excessive menstruation; Croupose—resembling croup; Bronchopneumonia—Inflammation of the lungs; Atypical fever—irregular fever; Dyspnoe—Hard breathing; Cyanosis—Blue discoloration of the skin from non-oxidation of the blood; Pleuritis—Pleurisy; Phthisis—consumption; Myocarditis and Endocarditis—Inflammations of the heart; Thrombosis—coagulation of blood; Intestinal Catarrh—Inflammation of the bowels; Dyspepsia—Indigestion; Neuritis—Nerve inflammation; Psychosis—Mental derangement; Otitis media—Inflammation of the ear; and Nephritis—Inflammation of the kidneys.

"Aetiology:—The influenza bacillus (found in blood and excrement) is to be regarded as the cause. The malady is highly contagious. Period of incubation given as, from two to seven days. Runs its course in one or two weeks, recovery as a rule favorable; though convalescence is often protracted. Unfavorable results are brought on through complications, most often by Pneumonia.

"Diagnosis:—Easily determined during an epidemic or marked symptoms. The catarrhal form of influenza differs from simple catarrh of the mucous membranes of the respiratory tract through the presence of nervous symptoms and a more abrupt beginning. The symptoms may be similar to those of Measles or Abdominal typhus. In each case, complications with Pneumonia must be considered.

"The proof of the presence of the Influenza bacillus," he concludes, "is of little value in the diagnosis and differential diagnosis in medical practice as the bacillus cannot be distinguished with enough accuracy through the microscopic examination, which must be a very minute culture proceeding."

This is the final dictum of medical Science on the subject—Science which however, adds nothing to our knowledge and leaves us still in darkness and uncertainty, while memory brings a well known couplet to the mind:

> He holds the threads of Wisdom's way
> Loosely, with palsied hand.
> Why lacks he now, for pity's sake,
> The grace to understand?

M.B.

(After Goethe.)

But let us weigh this long list of symptoms and estimate their respective significance by the light of physiological perception.

The ever present fever is due to stagnation of the blood. Swelling of the spleen is caused by catabolism of the Malpighian bodies. Albuminuria is the result of cold in the Plexus renalis; Perspiration is due to numbness in the nerve fibrils. The inclination of the mucous membranes to Hemorrhage is explained by congestion of blood in the capillaries, due to lack of vigor in the nerve fibrils. When the nerve fibrils fail to act, the capillary circulation stops and the blood overloaded with carbonic acid presses against the walls until they burst.

The complications and after effects are explained in the following manner:

Complications in the respiratory system are all due to failure to properly treat the acute stage of the disease, and where the resistance of the patient has been sapped they usually end fatally. Complications in the circulatory system are subject to the same explanation as fever. Digestive complications are due to impaired metabolism brought on by loss of energy in the Vagus nerve. Complications in the nervous system are consequent upon the degeneration of the whole Vagus tract. Sensory complications are due to the disease attacking the "minoris resistentia," the point of least resistance in the patient.

This explanation of the real significance of the symptoms of Influenza should make it sufficiently apparent that its cause is fundamental, widespread and deeply rooted in the organism — a menace not to be lightly and tentatively treated with impunity. That the disease is not one that may be met — with any prospect of success — with febrifuges, drugs, serums and specifics — to say nothing of whisky and the like futilities, to use no harsher term, such as are said to have characterized the prescriptions of a very considerable proportion of the Regular Medical Profession and with such terribly disastrous results. What the liquor statistics show on our side of the line I am at the moment unable to say, but I see it reported in the press of an adjoining province that under nominally strict "Prohibition" the sale of liquor had increased no less than 900 per cent, largely upon doctors orders, and that the sales from the Government stores in one city, during the past month had totaled $50,000 — as compared with $6,000 for the corresponding period of the previous year.

The Professor's elaborate diagnosis, from a physiologico-chemical point of view seems rather to point to a meaning which he has missed — to indicate a latent, more remote possibility behind the shy bacillus, as the primary cause of the disease.

Let us endeavor to read the riddle rightly. On scientific contemplation it at once becomes apparent that the symptoms as defined by Kuhnemann — and indeed all other observers — are confined to the regions traversed by the *Vagus* (wandering) or *Pneumogastric* nerve — a nerve of comprehensive scope and bi-functional activity, *physical and psychic* and in operation, remarkably in accord with the manifestations of Influenza.

Concisely stated, the physiological function of the *Vagus nerve* is to regulate the process of breathing, tasting, swallowing, appetite, digestion, etc.; and the result of its failure to function would create coughing, choking, indigestion—separately or in combination. Its mental functions include the expression of shame, desire, disgust, grief, torture, depression and despair.

The following is its academic description:

Vagus or Pneumogastric nerve (tenth cranial); function—sensation and motion; originates in the floor of the fourth ventricle (the space which represents the primitive cavity of the hind-brain; it has the pons and oblongata in front, while the cerebellum lies dorsal), and is distributed through the ear, pharynx, larynx, lungs, esophagus, and stomach; possesses the following branches—auricular, pharyngeal, superior and inferior laryngeal, cardiac, pulmonary, esophageal, gastric, hepatic, communicating, meningeal.

It is interesting to compare the scope and characteristics of the Vagus, as here defined with the details of Prof. Kuhnemann's diagnosis of Influenza and to draw conclusions.

In order to establish more unmistakably the symptomatic sympathetic connection between the Vagus and Influenza, it may be well to touch briefly upon the initial processes of metabolism and nerve production.

An inherent impulse in the ovum (protoplasm or egg cell) serves to separate the albuminous substance into groups of an opposite nature. Water is chemically separated from one portion, which results in thickening the albumen from which it was extracted, while the liberated water aids in liquifying another portion of the albuminous matter. Thus, on one side slender threads arise, termed fibrine or filaments, and on the other lymph fluid appears, which receives the particles of salts freed from the filaments during their chemical separation. When the fibrine and lymph are organized from the protoplasm, the remaining albumen is absolutely unchanged and ready to furnish material for the growth of either.

It is the function of salts to increase the electrical tension of the lymph. All salts possess the property of being electrically positive or negative. The more concentrated a saline solution, the greater its electrical energy.

That the function of the lymph is to assist in the formation and nutrition of the nerves is apparent when the nature of lymph and the composition of nerve substances are compared. The contrast which exists between fibrine and lymph, and the similarity of lymph to nerve fat when taken together, justify the conclusion that the nerve substance lecithin, was formed from lymph in the first instance.

The whole process of life consists of an electro-chemical combustion. This is clearly shown in the case of lecithin, which serves to control both motion and sensation. In the presence of oxygen it burns up, forming a new chemical combination, and throwing off minute quantities of carbonic acid and water in the process. *Every movement and process, both voluntary and involuntary, and every thought and emotion, depends upon oxidation, which consumes muscular tissue and nerve substance.*

The greater our physical exertion the more muscular tissue must be consumed. The higher our emotional state, the more we think or agitate ourselves, the greater must be the quantity of nerve substance burned up. All of the substance burned up in labour, in worry and in thought, must be replaced or the flame will flicker out!

The metabolism of muscular tissue is not in question at the moment. We are concerned here with nerve metabolism alone.

This occurs in the following manner: In response to the demand for new material created by the chemical combustion of lecithin, new oil flows down the axis cylinders of the nerve fibrils, which are arranged somewhat in the manner of lamp wicks. The average duration of the flow of this oil is about eighteen hours. When the cerebro-spinal nerves refuse to perform their function any longer, because the supply of oil is running low, fatigue and sleep ensue, and the blood descends from the brain to the intestines. Thus the cerebro-spinal system is permitted to relax and rest. In the meantime the sympathetic nervous system has taken up the task of directing the renewal of worn tissues, which draw their supply of necessary materials from the digestive canal, with a new supply of phosphatic oil. For the carrying out of these processes, which prepare the brain and spinal nerve system for the demands of another day, the magnetic blood current acts as distributor of supplies.

Through the fact that this supply is directly dependent upon nutrition, three possibilities inevitably present themselves:

(1) That any radical change of diet may result in an insufficient supply of the various elements necessary for the production of lecithin in the requisite quantities.

(2) That strenuous and unaccustomed physical and mental exertion may involve a consumption both of nerve substance and muscular tissue, greater than the outcome of the ordinary diet is able to compensate.

(3) That a protracted term of emotional strain and agitation may adversely affect both appetite and digestion while rapidly consuming the substance of the nerves.

In discussing the causes of disease Julius Hensel lays great stress upon the emotions. He goes so far as to say that they "*undoubtedly occupy the first place amongst the factors causing disease*, and we must not evade the consideration of them. *We shall find that their action also amounts to an electro-chemical process.*" I would not for an instant be understood to contend that the emotions alone are sufficient to explain the origin of disease—not at all. There are other factors—jointly or severally dominant—diet, occupation, changes of weather, climate, or conditions.

In the matter immediately under review, however, the world-wide pandemic of "Spanish Influenza," there can remain no shadow of doubt in the mind of any unbiased observer who follows the question fairly along the lines of electro-chemical biology, but that the general emotional disturbances incident upon the war conditions of the world, combined with the chaotic dietetic position with its anxieties and privations under strenuous and unwonted physical demands, do undoubtedly afford a sound and reasonable explanation of the cataclysmal outbreak which has recently fallen upon the nations.

The brazen blast of war, in 1914, with all its ruthless wreck and carnage, shook the universal fabric of the sphere. Fear, fraud and famine were met together, duplicity and greed had kissed each other. Short rations and with some, starvation, were soon the order of the day. The corners of the earth were swept of stale forgotten stores and profiteers waxed fat and prices soared, whilst the vitals of the working world were vastly underfed. The ranks of labour, depleted of its men, were filled by females uninured to toil and dangerous nerve racking environments. Relentless time brings its revenges fast; but still they worked and suffered while malnutrition sapped the life-blood of the race. In the homes of the fighting men fear reigned supreme—ever the sword of Damocles suspended at the hearth. And then the death lists came and the world was wet with human tears and all the furies flew the earth—grief, hatred, revenge, love, pity and remorse, but the wail of mourning was throughout all lands in all the "sable panoply of woe" attending fast lowering vitality, bred by force of pain and hope deferred. Pliny well said: "Dolendi modus, non est timendi"—Pain has its limits, *apprehension none*—and now as in his day, the latter bore the palm.

Such was the position when two years ago the world first felt the impact of the pestilence and millions withered up like blighted corn.

The Vagus nerve with which we have been dealing, is concerned with the expression of emotions such as these; and being so, was burned up rapidly with fervent heat—the flames of sorrow still with fasting fed. In the majority of human lives such was the case, while the sources of nutritive reserve force were depleted by lack of things of universal use and foreign substitutes for normal food. Small wonder then the once steady nerves soon buckled with the strain; that sickness followed swiftly with disaster in its train and that the death rate rose enormously, beyond recorded precedent. And then when seeming good succeeds the storm of ills a plethora of new-born cares arose and worse, more fatal still, reaction from the strain which with relaxing energy demands its deadly share. Here in America we meet our troubles with serener front, unawed by State-fed sacerdotal superstitions; but in England how the scourge has wrung from dire depression its full toll of death. There for the first time deaths exceed the births and for the final quarter of 1918, the deaths exceed those of the former term by 127,000 of which Influenza claimed one hundred Thousand dead. Similar conditions, it would appear, have been more or less general throughout the European and indeed all other Continents and the title "Pandemic" has been richly earned; but the term which would seem to me more descriptive still would be "*Panasthenia*" – *the general loss of vitality*.

The human organism is, as we know, electro-magnetic. The effect upon the fabric of abnormal disturbance is registered with infinite exactitude by electrons—atoms of electricity—which rise and fall in numerical vibration according to the positive or negative tone of the whole; and excessive manifestations in one direction or the other, indicate respectively, a condition of positive or negative disease.

When the slowly vibrating negative electrons outnumber the rapidly vibrating positive atoms the electronic vibration of the whole body is lowered. As a result, we become depressed, weak, tired and retain little bodily warmth. Digestion is upset, metabolism falls far below normal, and the skin becomes pale, because of the morbid action set up in the mucous membrane by the excess of negative electrons. Catarrh supervenes. This is the condition in which negative disease thrives best: Influenza, nervous debility, anaemia, sleeping disease, cholera, diphtheria and the rest, in all varied forms of negative disease.

The Vagus, or Wandering Nerve, permeates every vital section of the body, as the accompanying plate will show. It controls, as has been shown, all the highest functions, both mental and physical of human life—that life which depends for its well-being upon electro-chemical combustion, metabolism, and the fuel supply we designate as food. It is the first postulate of healthy vitality in the human frame that metabolism and catabolism—intake and output—shall go hand in hand—that the body must receive continually such fresh nutrition as may replace what it consumes in the process of muscular action and the exercise of mental and emotional activity, and we are consequently brought to the conclusion that such bonds of safety and provision being rudely and suddenly severed, all physical resistance must be quickly broken down, the latent reserve energy is used and disappears, psychic resolution—the immunity of mind—soon abdicates its throne and the depleted organism, robbed of all defense, falls victim to contagion when it comes to kill.

Treatment.

As regards the treatment, actual and preventive, applicable to Spanish Influenza, the methods employed under the Hygienic-Dietetic System of Healing have been already defined in a previous chapter on the subject of negative disease in general. Instruction, however, devoted to Influenza alone may be found in Chapter VI of the special pamphlet issued in that connection under the title: "Influenza, Cause and Cure," [E] and also in my greater work: "Regeneration or Dare to be Healthy," now in course of completion.

And now, one final word in conclusion, for the purpose of drawing together, as it were, the multiplicity of threads which constitute the complex skein of causes and effects, with their remedial measures which cover the wide range of human life's vicissitudes—the interruptions of its would-be harmonies—which take the forms, all too common in these times of stress, of physical disturbance and of mental strain which come to us in the combined and threatening guise of suffering and disease.

That these forms are more pronounced, more virulent today than ever before in the records of the race, is surely great Nature's manner, crude and masterful, of pressing her mandate home—right home upon the plastic film of evanescent shadows and ephemeral shades we proudly call our consciousness.

How many, let me ask, how many of us, in the absorbing round of life's futilities, have paused to really recognize the sinister "hand writing on the wall?"

The phase of the world's history through which we pass complacently is of no light portent, its happenings no casual concern, but, in point of crucial fact, a virtual "rending of the sphere"—a cosmic upheaval such as never yet before has racked the tense life sinews of the world, confounding the wisdom of the wise and wrecking in one fell climax of contempt the moral precepts of two thousand years.

The greatest human struggle the world has ever known synchronizes strangely, yet logically with the world's greatest pestilence which has swept successive millions to their doom without exacting from the residue even the sentimental tribute of a tear.

The official brains of the entire globe are leagued in self-protective unison "to make the world safe for democracy;" but Demos dies, by violence and disease, ere yet salvation comes. It appeals to its old-time standards for relief,—they are gone; to its pastors—they are mute; to its masters—they are impotent; to its doctors—they are baffled, helpless and aghast, whilst vainly searching earth and air for some frail pretext of unreal enlightenment, some fragile figment of belief. And yet in hypnotized complacency the masses stand; for meanwhile commerce reaps its costly gains and labour draws in enhanced increment the wages of the living and the dead.

Less serious visitations have, in former times, left their eternal imprint on the age. They served to point the moral of widespread reform—to emphasize the practice of hygiene and sanity. For all such scourges are but signs of Nature's trust betrayed, her sacred laws defied in the wild rush for gain, oblivious of the Law of Compensation's cost, with its inevitable reckoning.

Thus, to the discoverer of the lost initiative, what prospect does the future hold in store?

Pandemics, such as this, repeat themselves; and other forms of dread disease are following the footsteps of mankind. Arterio sclerosis, (hardening of the arteries), with its kindred complaints, for instance, now threatens to become a standing feature of the race through ignorance of the physiological functions of the nerves, their tissue exhaustion and supply.

With such impending dangers are our men distressed; and yet there seems but grudging, slight encouragement for those who seek to stay the onslaught of the foe, by scientific measures of precaution and hygiene.

What the nation needs is now a practical and nation-wide awakening. Let the people realize the danger of their risk; let them rally to the call and loyally support those who thus offer them the safeguard of knowledge as a refuge from the impending storm. Then will so-called "incurable disease" be relegated to the limbo of the past and, among other prophylactic means, this, my latest great discovery—the cause of Influenza, its prevention and its cure, a discovery which must rank amongst the great scientific achievements of the day—will mitigate the force of epidemics on mankind. It should also give to the reader of this little book a fair assurance of what immunity it is possible to secure by careful study and practice of its truths and should prove to the thinker the nucleus of a lesson which can nowhere be better learned than in the teachings and the precepts of the Hygienic-Dietetic School.

> "But to the hero, when his sword
> Has won the battle for the free,
> Thy voice sounds like a prophet's word
> And in its hollow tones are heard
> The thanks of millions yet to be"

FINIS.

Wide and unlimited as the field of biology and the hygienic-dietetic method of healing is, I have in the foregoing pages tried to devise a guide that will indicate the points that are most necessary to the confidence of the patient, based upon knowledge.

If I have enlightened my readers sufficiently regarding the most modern results of biological research, if I have succeeded in showing them the ray of hope, in the midst of their suffering, that will give them courage to live, and live as healthy human beings, I shall feel amply rewarded for the hard work that had necessarily to be done before the present pinnacle in the art of healing could be reached.

Let me repeat: this brochure is not designed to lead any one away from the man who knows, who has gone to the sources of wisdom, to bring salvation to those who demand the right to live in health and vigor. Far otherwise; for my deliberate injunction is that the cure of disease, in any form, should not be undertaken except under the guidance of an hygienic physician who may indicate to them the path, so that they may not tread it blindly, but in the light of knowledge.

The outlines of a great and wonderful science are presented. Another wall between the layman and the professional has been torn down. If, my readers, you can one day say this booklet has guided you to the right path, back to the enjoyment of life in youthful health and vigor, then join with me and others in propagating these sane and safe principles, and make others "Dare to be Healthy," as you have dared yourself.

FOOTNOTES:

[D] This amount is given by the Seattle Post-Intelligencer, in an editorial devoted to the terrible plague on March 16th, 1919.

[E] The pamphlet, which also contains a chart of the Vagus in 2 colors, may be obtained either from the author or through any bookseller. The price is 50 cents.